UPGRADE YOUR IMMUNITY
WITH HERBS

ALSO BY DR. JOSEPH MERCOLA

EMF'D*

KetoFast Cookbook (with Pete Evans)*

KetoFast*

Fat for Fuel Ketogenic Cookbook (with Pete Evans)*

Fat for Fuel*

Effortless Healing

The No-Grain Diet

Take Control of Your Health

Sweet Deception

Dark Deception

The Great Bird Flu Hoax

Freedom at Your Fingertips

Generation XL

Healthy Recipes for Your Nutritional Type

*Available from Hay House

Please visit:

Hay House USA: www.hayhouse.com®
Hay House Australia: www.hayhouse.com.au
Hay House UK: www.hayhouse.co.uk
Hay House India: www.hayhouse.co.in

UPGRADE YOUR IMMUNITY
WITH HERBS

HERBAL TONICS, BROTHS, BREWS, AND ELIXIRS TO SUPERCHARGE YOUR IMMUNE SYSTEM

Dr. Joseph Mercola

HAY HOUSE, INC.
Carlsbad, California | New York City
London | Sydney | New Delhi

Published in the United States by: Hay House, Inc.: www.hayhouse.com®
Published in Australia by: Hay House, Inc.: www.hayhouse.com.au
Published in the United Kingdom by: Hay House UK, Ltd.: www.hayhouse.co.uk
Published in India by: Hay House Publishers India: www.hayhouse.co.in

Cover design: Scott Breidenthal • *Interior design:* Bryn Starr Best
Interior photos: William Meppem, Mark Roper, and Steve Brown
Food stylists: Lucy Tweed and Deborah Kaloper
Images used under license from Shutterstock.com: Pages 15–16, 23–24, 33–34
Indexer: J S Editorial, LLC

Cataloging-in-Publication Data is on file at the Library of Congress

Names: Mercola, Joseph, author.
Title: Upgrade your immunity with herbs : herbal tonics, broths, brews, and elixirs to supercharge your immune system / Dr. Joseph Mercola.
Description: 1st edition. | Carlsbad, California : Hay House, Inc., 2021. |
    Identifiers: LCCN 2021005515 | ISBN 9781401963484 (hardback) | ISBN 9781401963491 (ebook)
Subjects: LCSH: Herbs--Therapeutic use. | Naturopathy--Popular works.
Classification: LCC RM666.H33 M4437 2021 | DDC 615.3/21--dc23
LC record available at https://lccn.loc.gov/2021005515

Hardcover ISBN: 978-1-4019-6348-4
E-book ISBN: 978-1-4019-6349-1
Audiobook ISBN: 978-1-4019-6353-8

10 9 8 7 6 5 4 3 2 1
1st edition, May 2021

Printed in the United States of America

SUSTAINABLE FORESTRY INITIATIVE
Certified Chain of Custody
Promoting Sustainable Forestry
www.sfiprogram.org
SFI-01268
SFI label applies to the text stock

CONTENTS

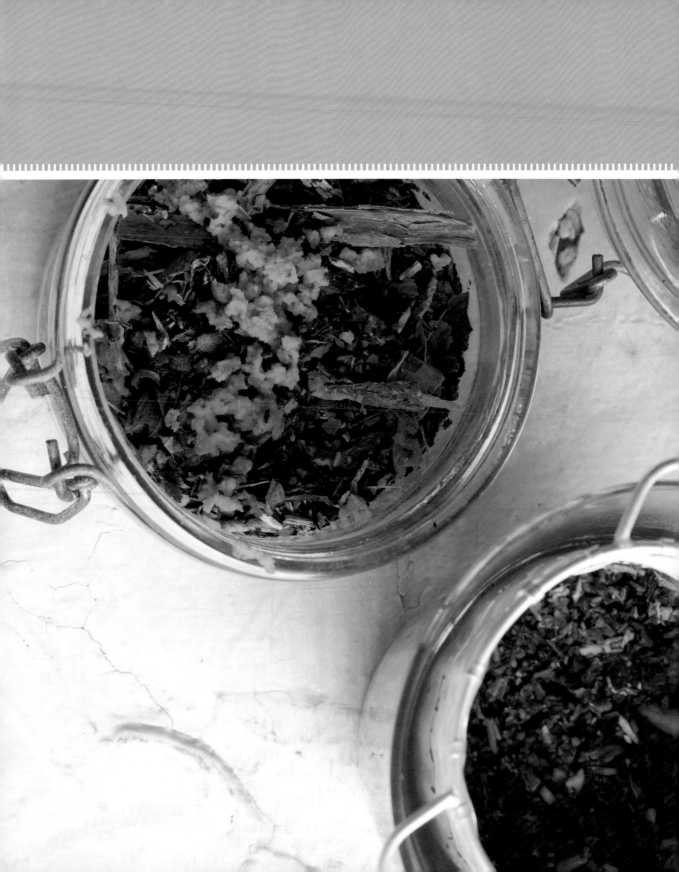

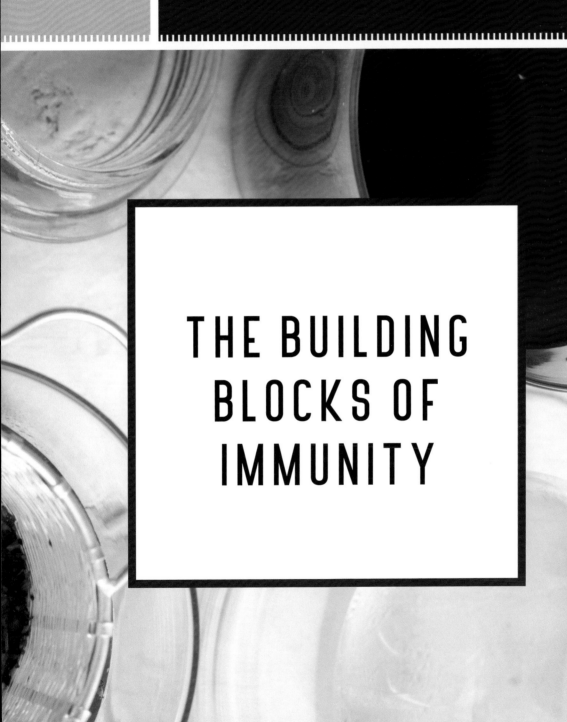

PART I

THE BUILDING BLOCKS OF IMMUNITY

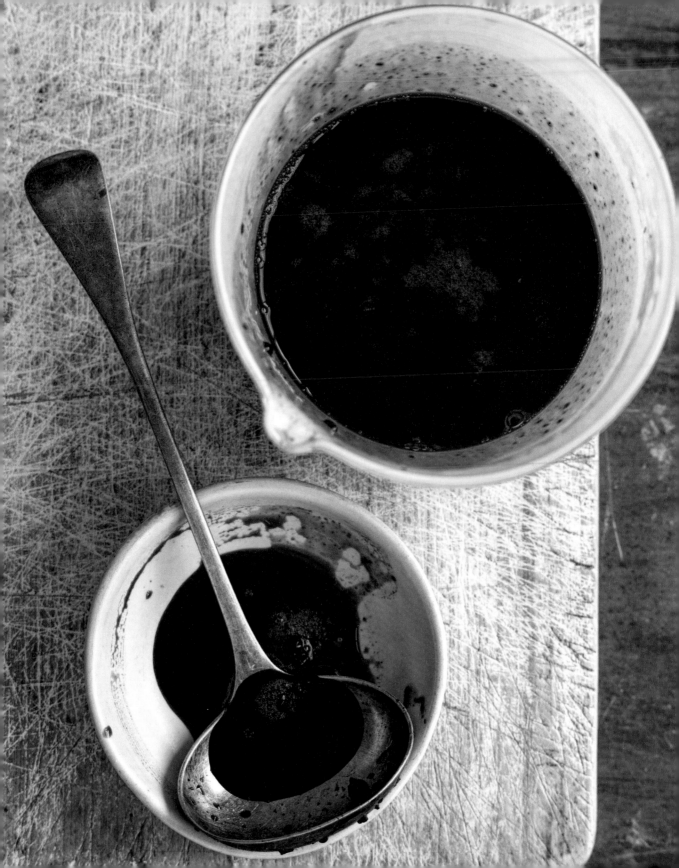

Your immune system is your first line of defense against all disease, especially infectious disease, and there are many different ways to boost your immune system and improve its function.

Think of your immune system as an army whose primary job is to protect you from invaders. Just like an army, you want your immune system to be responsive; to be able to correctly discern what is a threat and what isn't; to use the appropriate force to neutralize the enemy without causing collateral damage; and to have the stamina to keep fighting until the danger has receded.

What you *don't* want is to have your immune system launch such a massive response that it harms your tissues—as is the case with the storm of cytokines (particularly potent immune cells) that COVID-19 triggers in a small percentage of cases. Or to always be on high alert with chronic inflammation. Or for your body to become its own enemy, as it does with autoimmune conditions.

A healthy immune system is balanced. It can ramp up, and it can stand at ease. While there are medicines designed to stimulate your immune system and others to suppress it, what you really want is a highly functioning, balanced immune system, one that doesn't rely on medications or the actions of others to protect you.

The Three Types of Immunity

As I write this book, we are in the throes of the COVID-19 pandemic, and many people are waiting for a magical vaccine to provide widespread immunity to the virus so we can safely resume living our lives and enjoying shared space with people once again. There are a few flaws in this thinking:

- The best way to develop immunity to any infectious threat is through natural exposure. Although it carries a risk of getting sick, natural exposure is what helps you develop a broader immunity both to a specific virus and to all pathogens as your immune system grows stronger from use. It's a paradox of the human body that getting sick is the best thing to prevent you from getting sick.

- Your immune system has two branches—the cellular (T cells) and the humoral (B cells)—and both need to be activated in order to secure long-term immunity. When you get a vaccine, you stimulate only your humoral immunity, the B cells. The T cells are not stimulated.

It's important to know that even the medications and vaccines that so many rely on for protection against disease don't work by themselves; they work by supporting your immune system so that it can better defend against whatever particular threat the vaccine is designed to overcome. So no medicine is a savior; ultimately, that role falls to your own immune system. And the stronger it is, the stronger you are.

For these reasons, it makes far more sense to optimize your immune system's function so you can withstand whatever pathogens you're exposed to and develop what's known as active immunity, which is one of the three basic types of immunity and also the best and longest lasting. The three types are:

- **Active immunity,** which comes from the actions your immune system takes to protect you from pathogens. It is the result of your immune system fighting off a threat. Thanks to your immune system's ability to remember how to fight invaders it has already encountered, in most cases, active immunity lasts a lifetime.

    This immunologic memory comes thanks to T cells and B cells, which retain the ability to recognize and fight every particular pathogen they encounter. These two types of immune cells circulate at low levels until they identify a familiar pathogen. Then they rise in level and trigger other immune cells to ramp up their defenses too.

- **Passive immunity,** which is passed along via immunity gained by someone else. For example, a pregnant mother can pass antibodies to her unborn child through her placenta, or through her breast milk once the baby is born. Passive immunity can also be transferred through immunoglobulin treatments, where antibodies that have been developed by individuals who have fought off that pathogen are injected into someone who hasn't. Although passive immunity can be lifesaving, it is short lived, because those antibodies don't get stored in immunologic memory.

- **Community immunity,** otherwise known as herd immunity. This occurs when individuals are protected by the people around them. This does not involve the protected person's immune system at all. Rather, it relies on the immune systems of others. In herd immunity, when enough people have developed immunity to a particular pathogen, the virus has fewer people it can infect and thus, fewer potential carriers. As a result, there are fewer outbreaks and fewer instances of infection.

    You can also create community immunity by a process called cocooning—which is making sure that a vulnerable person shares close personal space only with healthy individuals. This is the tactic many took with their elders or immunocompromised loved ones when the COVID-19 pandemic struck. Because herd immunity doesn't build immunologic memory, it is the least reliable form of immunity.

By far, the best choice is to cultivate your active immunity. When you strengthen your own immune system, you strengthen your ability to create active immunity. You also contribute to herd immunity as you remove yourself from the possible pool of people who can spread a particular pathogen, making it less likely that those who don't have immunity will be exposed to it.

As COVID-19 has shown us, it is absolutely essential to strengthen our immune systems, as it is inevitable that we will all be exposed to not only the novel coronavirus but also other viruses.

The good news is that your immune system has a long history of working to protect you against myriad threats. It is adaptable and resilient. To optimize it, you simply need to provide it with optimal nutrition and avoid toxic exposures. This cookbook is a practical resource to help you do just that. And the recipes in Part II make it delicious to do so. All of the recipes incorporate the immune-boosting herbs and foods I cover in Part I—some consist primarily of a specific herb (like a ginger tea that you brew and drink), while some are part of a delicious meal (for example, a sautéed lamb dish that puts garlic front and center).

While my focus is on showing you how to use nature's medicine cabinet of herbs and spices to give your immune system a boost, I'll also cover the basics of robust immunity; sleep hygiene; proper hydration; a healthy diet that includes a wide range of essential nutrients, vitamins, and antioxidants; and gut health.

The herbs, spices, and health-promoting practices you'll encounter on these pages will help you resist diseases of all types, whether it's a novel infectious disease like COVID-19 or something chronic like diabetes, Alzheimer's, or cancer.

They will also help you become more resilient to the *fear* of getting sick, because you'll know how to give your immune system what it needs to function well. And getting over fear is how you become empowered to take care of everything in your life, including your health.

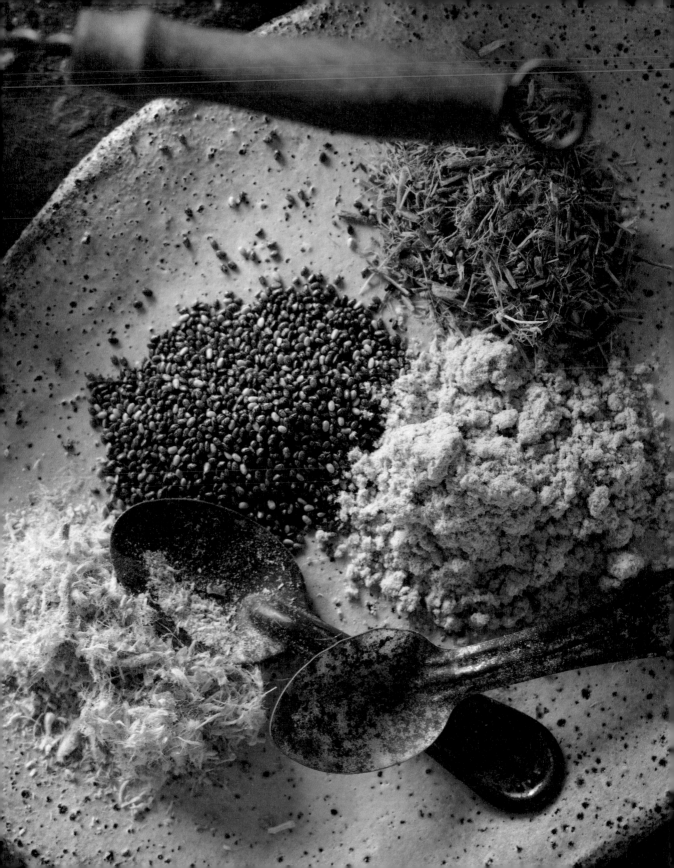

Before the advent of drugs, plant remedies were the go-to medicines. Although science and technology have advanced to the point where most of our medicines are now created in labs, the benefits of herbs and spices haven't changed. They can serve you just as well today as they served your ancestors in the past.

One of the reasons that herbs and spices are immune supportive is that they are some of the foods richest in antioxidants. Many herbs and spices top the list of high-ORAC-value foods. ORAC stands for *oxygen radical absorbance capacity* and is a standardized method of measuring the antioxidant capacity of different foods and supplements. The higher the ORAC score, the more effective a food is at neutralizing harmful free radicals, which are highly unstable molecules that lack an electron. Free radicals damage other, healthy molecules in search of a replacement to their missing electron. The fewer free radicals available to attack your cells and tissues, the more your immune system can focus on fighting external invaders and keeping your whole system in balance, or what's called homeostasis.

Scoring high on the ORAC scale isn't the only reason why herbs and spices pack such a powerful punch. They're also very dense in nutrients such as vitamins and minerals, many of which are vital players in immunity (and which I'll cover in the next section).

Additionally, herbs and spices have medicinal properties. This should come as no surprise considering they've been used as medicine for thousands of years prior to the advent of modern medicine that focuses on synthetic drugs in lieu of these natural counterparts.

Each herb and spice has a unique set of health benefits to offer. As a general rule, it is hard to go wrong when using herbs and spices. I recommend adding fresh, organic herbs and spices to all your meals, allowing your taste buds to dictate your choices when cooking. However, herbs are such powerful medicine that you should also find ways beyond your daily meals to ingest them. That's what this cookbook is designed to help you do. It will show you how many avenues you have to fine-tune your immunity through teas, tonics, jams, and juices in addition to your meals.

Eating a wide array of herbs and spices on a regular basis can go a long way toward preventing chronic illness. Herbs favorably impact your health in a variety of ways:

- **Boosting your body's immune response.** Take garlic, for example. This kitchen staple delivers its benefits on multiple levels, offering antibacterial, antiviral, antifungal, and antioxidant properties. A 2019 review and meta-analysis of earlier research concluded that garlic effectively lowered several inflammatory biomarkers, including C-reactive protein, TNF-α, and interleukin-6.[1] It's thought that much of garlic's therapeutic effects come from its sulfur-containing compounds, such as allicin. Research has revealed that as your body digests allicin it produces sulfenic acid, a compound that reacts faster with dangerous free radicals than any other known compound.[2]

And that's just one example. Every herb and spice contains multiple components that can each play a role in supporting your immunity—unlike pharmaceuticals derived from herbs, which typically contain only one or two primary constituents. They also work synergistically to influence one another and extend their benefits in ways science is only beginning to understand.

- **Fighting cancer.** As I mentioned in the introduction, herbs and spices help to protect you from not just infectious diseases, but also the chronic diseases that claim so many lives and diminish quality of life for many others. These include perhaps the scariest disease of them all—cancer. There are three herbal constituents in particular that have demonstrated cancer-fighting abilities, including:

    o **Apigenin.** This flavonoid (a category of phytochemicals that give plants their pigments and offer an array of health benefits) is found in many herbs, including parsley, thyme, and chamomile, as well as in certain other plants and vegetables, such as celery. It has been widely established that apigenin is important for brain health, and it is hailed for its anticancer abilities. When mice implanted with cells of a particularly deadly and fast-growing human breast cancer were treated with apigenin, the cancerous growth slowed and the tumors shrank. Blood vessels feeding the tumors also shrank and restricted blood flow to the tumor cells, starving them of the nutrients needed to spread.[3] Interestingly, the compound was also found to bind to 160 proteins in the human body, which suggests it has far-reaching health effects—unlike pharmaceutical drugs, which typically have only one specific target.

    Apigenin is a component of chamomile tea, and may even be one reason why drinking chamomile tea has been found to reduce thyroid cancer risk by up to 80 percent.[4]

    o **Curcumin.** This primary constituent of turmeric has more evidence to back up its anticancer claims than any other nutrient. In India, where turmeric is widely used, the prevalence of four common cancers—colon, breast, prostate, and lung—is one-tenth as high as it is in the United States. Specifically, curcumin has been found to:

- Inhibit the transformation of cells from normal to tumor, as well as inhibit the proliferation of tumor cells already existing
- Help the body destroy mutated cancer cells so they cannot spread throughout the body
- Decrease inflammation
- Enhance liver function
- Inhibit the synthesis of a protein thought to be instrumental in tumor formation
- Prevent the development of additional blood supply necessary for cancer cell growth (known as anti-angiogenesis)

o **Ashwagandha.** This traditional Indian herb is packed with flavonoids that lend it many powerful properties. In one study, bioactive withanolides—naturally occurring steroids—in ashwagandha were identified as agents that suppress pathways responsible for several inflammation-based illnesses, including arthritis, asthma, hypertension, osteoporosis, and cancer.[5]

Ashwangandha is what's known as an adaptogen, which can either stimulate or suppress your immune system to help fight infections, cancer, and other diseases, as well as help relieve the mental and physical effects of stress. There are many other adaptogenic herbs, including ginseng and rhodiola (which are covered in depth on pages 25 and 35, respectively). Their ability to provide just what's needed and restore balance is evidence of the wisdom of nature.

- **Combating medical conditions.** In addition, numerous herbs and spices do a lot of heavy lifting in addressing medical conditions that so many suffer from, including:

o **Alzheimer's disease.** Curcumin has been found to inhibit the accumulation of destructive beta amyloids in the brain of Alzheimer's patients, as well as to break up existing plaques.[6] In fact, it is more effective in inhibiting the formation of these protein fragments than many other potential Alzheimer's treatments.

People with Alzheimer's tend to have higher levels of inflammation in their brains, and curcumin is best known for its potent anti-inflammatory properties. The compound has been shown to influence the expression of more than 700 genes, and it can inhibit both the activity and the synthesis of many enzymes that modulate inflammation.

o **Diabetes.** The popular spice cinnamon is a powerful modulator of blood sugar. It helps diabetics deal with insulin sensitivity and glucose transport, and it decreases inflammation. In one study, 18 people with type 2 diabetes participated in a 12-week trial in which half the group took 1,000 milligrams (mg) of cassia cinnamon supplements and the other half took a placebo. According to the study conclusion, all the subjects in the cinnamon group had a statistically significant decrease in their blood sugar levels (comparable to oral medications available for diabetes), while the placebo group had less positive results.[7]

- Blood pressure. High blood pressure can damage your heart and blood vessels by making them work harder and less efficiently. Over time, high blood pressure damages the inner lining of your arteries. It is often called "the silent killer" since symptoms are not usually noticeable. Nearly half of all adults in the United States now have high blood pressure.

  In one study researchers tested olive leaf extract as a food supplement in a group of 40 identical twins who had borderline high blood pressure. One twin in each pair received olive leaf extract for eight weeks, while the other received advice on changing lifestyle factors that impact blood pressure. Every two weeks the researchers measured the group's body weight, blood pressure, heart rate, glucose, and lipids. In those who received the olive leaf extract, the dose was 500 or 1,000 mg per day.

The researchers found a change in blood pressure that appeared to be dependent on the dose. In those receiving 500 mg, systolic pressure went down 6 mmHg more than it did in the control group. In those receiving 1,000 mg, systolic pressure went down 13 mmHg. After eight weeks, the average blood pressures in the control group were nearly identical to baseline, but they were significantly reduced in the group taking 1,000 mg.[8]

All these health benefits give you ample reason to be adventurous in adding spices to your meals, to be generous in the amounts you use, and to expand your repertoire of recipes to include more tonics, teas, and jams whose primary aim is to increase your herb consumption. Your efforts will be worth it for the flavor enhancement alone, and the boost it will give your health is the icing on the cake.

On the following pages, I'll give you a tour through the 19 herbs and spices that I believe to be the most important for immunity.

ANDROGRAPHIS

A proven immune booster used worldwide

What it is: Androgaphis—botanical name *Androgaphis paniculata*—is one of the most widely used medicinal plants across the globe. It's native to India and Sri Lanka and is also commonly found throughout China and Southeast Asia. Known as the "king of bitters" for its extremely acrid taste, it produces leaves, flowers, and roots that have been used for centuries to treat a variety of ailments and conditions, from snake bites, diarrhea, and fever to respiratory infection, diabetes, and even cancer. Andrographis has long been used in Ayurveda, India's traditional healing system, and is a well-known constituent in many Ayurvedic herbal formulas. In traditional Chinese medicine, it is regarded for its ability to rid the body of heat and dispel toxins.

What the science says: Numerous studies have evaluated the traditional claims and medicinal potential of andrographis. A wealth of lab and animal research indicates that the herb has immune-stimulating capabilities as well as anti-inflammatory, antimicrobial, antiviral, and anticancer properties. Human studies demonstrate some of this activity as well.

For instance, andrographis appears to reduce the severity of the common cold and may even help ward it off in the first place. One double-blind, placebo-controlled trial of 61 adults with a cold found that those given tablets made with the dried extract of andrographis for five days experienced significant clinical improvement on day four of the treatment.[9]

Likewise, in one study, healthy students given andrographis tablets for cold prevention had a 2.1 times higher prevention rate compared with those given a placebo.[10] Other, similar studies have also found the herb to relieve the upper respiratory symptoms associated with a cold and to help prevent the development of infection.

The herb appears to suppress the flu as well. In one lab study of nine medicinal plants, andrographis showed the most promise in inhibiting the influenza virus, specifically H1N1, with more than a 50 percent suppression effect.[11] Elsewhere, a randomized, controlled human study found that patients with an influenza diagnosis who were given a standardized extract of andrographis not only recovered more quickly than the control group but also experienced fewer post-flu complications.[12] These actions against cold and flu are thought to be, at least in part, due to the immune-enhancing effects of its active constituents, namely andrographolides.

What's more, the herb may enhance your body's own defenses against the proliferation or spread of cancer cells and even cause cancer cells to die. More than 20 years ago, lab testing showed andrographis to inhibit the growth of human breast cancer cells in a manner similar to that of the popular breast cancer drug tamoxifen.[13] Subsequent lab and animal research has evaluated its anticancer activity on gastric, colorectal, and other types of cancer cells. Scientists also believe, based on the well-documented immune-boosting activity of andrographis, that it might be effective in treating autoimmune diseases.

Try it: There is a wide variety of andrographis supplements on the market; you may find it in combination with other herbs as well, such as eleuthero and echinacea. I like using andrographis stems in a delicious tea (see page 67).

ASHWAGANDHA

An ancient adaptogen

What it is: Ashwagandha is revered in Ayurveda, India's ancient healing system. In fact, it's one of the most important and prominent herbs in Ayurvedic medicine. Considered a *rasayana*, or tonic, it's believed to have wide-ranging health benefits, with the capacity to positively affect multiple bodily systems, including the nervous, endocrine, and reproductive systems.

It's also categorized as an adaptogen, a group of herbs that help support the body's ability to handle—or adapt to—stress. Indeed, most rasayana herbs are adaptogens, as *rasayana* is defined as an herbal preparation that not only promotes physical and mental vitality but also expands happiness.

Ashwagandha is a Sanskrit word that translates to "smell of the horse." The herb is so named because its fresh roots are said to smell like the animal, and also because of its purported ability to increase strength to stallion-like levels. Its roots and leaves are often turned to for preparations, but the flowers and seeds of the small shrub (*Withania somnifera*) can be used as medicine as well. You may also hear the herb called Indian ginseng or winter cherry.

What the science says: The herb appears to bolster the immune system in a variety of ways. Research suggests that many of ashwagandha's biologically active constituents, especially those known as withanolides, have immune-modulating properties. Specifically, they improve your body's defenses against disease by boosting the action of immune cells, including lymphocytes known as natural killer (NK) cells, which help the body reject tumors and viruses. The herb's chemical components also have proven antioxidant properties that protect immune cells from damage by free radicals.

Ashwagandha's ability to improve resilience to stress is well documented, as is stress's capacity to impair the immune system and significantly weaken our armor to infection. In one 2019 randomized, placebo-controlled study, 58 male and female adults with a high level of perceived stress were split into three groups, with two groups receiving different doses of ashwagandha extract and one receiving a placebo.

Stress was assessed via a questionnaire and a blood test that measured levels of the stress hormone cortisol. Sleep quality was also evaluated—science shows that lack of sleep can also negatively impact immunity. The results indicated that treatment with ashwagandha was "considerably effective" compared with the placebo. Indeed, participants taking ashwagandha showed a statistically significant reduction in stress levels according to both the questionnaire and the blood test, along with significant improvement in sleep quality. Those taking the higher dose of the herb also experienced a significant reduction in anxiety.[14]

Try it: Ashwagandha can be purchased in capsules, as a tincture, or as a loose powder; you'll also see it in tea formulations. I like to have ashwagandha root powder on hand to combine with other relaxing herbs like chamomile and lavender in a dreamy sleep tonic (page 68).

ASTRAGALUS ROOT

Fundamental to Chinese herbology

What it is: *Huang qi*, otherwise known as astragalus, has been a mainstay of traditional Chinese medicine (TCM) for thousands of years. Its roots, and occasionally stem, are used widely in TCM to boost energy and immunity, as well as to treat conditions from anemia and allergies to fever and uterine concerns; proponents also cite its benefits for heart health. It's one of TCM's 50 fundamental herbs and an essential ingredient in more than 200 Chinese herbal formulations.

Astragalus was even mentioned in *The Divine Husbandman's Classic of Materia Medica*, a 2,000-year-old Eastern Han Dynasty text on medicinal substances. Sometimes also referred to as milk vetch, it comes from a flowering plant in the legume family. There are thousands of species of astragalus, but it's *Astragalus membranaceus* that's primarily found in herbal supplements.

What the science says: More than 200 chemical components of astragalus have been identified. An array of isoflavonoids and polysaccharides in particular appear to be responsible for astragalus's health benefits. Studies indicate these compounds may do everything from helping to regulate blood lipids and blood glucose to playing an anti-aging role in the body. A wealth of research, conducted primarily in the lab and in animals, has investigated their ability to strengthen the immune system specifically, and the results are promising.

In addition to helping improve immune-signaling pathways, which activate your body's innate immune response, it appears astragalus polysaccharides promote growth of immune cells, including NK cells (discussed in the section on Ashwagandha) and macrophages, which are large, specialized immune cells that recognize and destroy bacteria and harmful organisms. Research also indicates these polysaccharides help dendritic cells grow and mature; these cells are crucial in activating the immune response.

Moreover, the science shows that the herb's polysaccharides have various effects on cytokines, such as increasing the levels of cytokines that help signal your immune system to get to work and reducing pro-inflammatory cytokines that are destructive to health. In fact, a clinical study of patients whose cancer had spread to other parts of the body reported a significant reduction of cancer symptom clusters (two or more concurrent symptoms) and a reduction in the amount or activity of major pro-inflammatory cytokines within the first month after treatment with astragalus polysaccharides.[15]

Studies suggest that astragalus may also help children ward off upper respiratory tract infections and may play a critical role in immune regulation related to asthma.[16] Further, research indicates astragalus may be an immunosuppressive agent and thus may possibly serve as a treatment for certain autoimmune disorders.

Try it: Astragalus root is processed into different forms of supplements, including capsules, powders, teas, and liquid extracts. You can also buy whole astragalus root slices, which can be enjoyed in a rich and healthful broth (page 71).

CHYAWANPRASH

One powerful paste

What it is: Chyawanprash, sometimes spelled chyavanprash and commonly abbreviated CP, isn't an individual herb. Rather, it's a synergistic Ayurvedic blend of roughly 50 different herbs and spices, along with honey, ghee, and other ingredients. Together they form a potent paste. CP has been used since ancient times to boost immunity and increase longevity. The formula consists primarily of amla, or Indian gooseberry, a known immune booster that's said to be the world's richest source of vitamin C. It also contains ashwagandha and many other immune-stimulating herbs. Its taste is said to be sweet, sour, bitter, and astringent all at once.

What the science says: A number of individual herbs within the CP formulation have been studied for their effects on the immune system. For example, in addition to the wealth of research on ashwagandha, amla has been shown to have antioxidant and immune-modulating properties. Another component, guduchi, has been shown to possess immune-stimulating capabilities as well as antimicrobial, anti-inflammatory, and antioxidant effects—and specifically to play a "substantial therapeutic role" in defending your body from salmonella poisoning.[17]

CP as a whole has also been evaluated for its effects on immunity, with research suggesting it increases the number and activity of immune cells and reduces the chance of infection. Notably, in a six-month clinical study in children ages 5 to 12, CP led to "significant improvement" in immunity as well as energy level, strength and physical fitness, and quality of life. When compared with the control group, children taking CP showed more than two times the protection from immunity-related illness (episodes of allergy conditions and infections).[18]

Interestingly, one experimental study showed that pretreatment with CP in rodents helped their systems experience lower histamine levels when they were then exposed to allergens. The researchers also found that the animals experienced an increase in NK cells and other powerful immune cells.[19] In general, studies support CP's use to improve the immunity and function of the respiratory system, citing its ability to help treat issues from asthma to tuberculosis.

Try it: The herbal blend is available from many online outlets and can be taken by the spoonful.

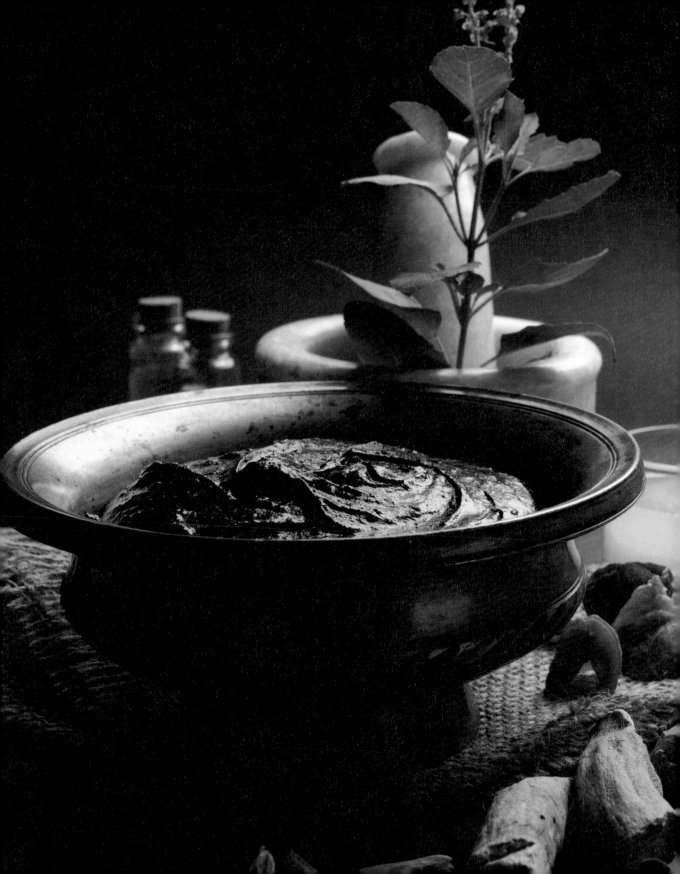

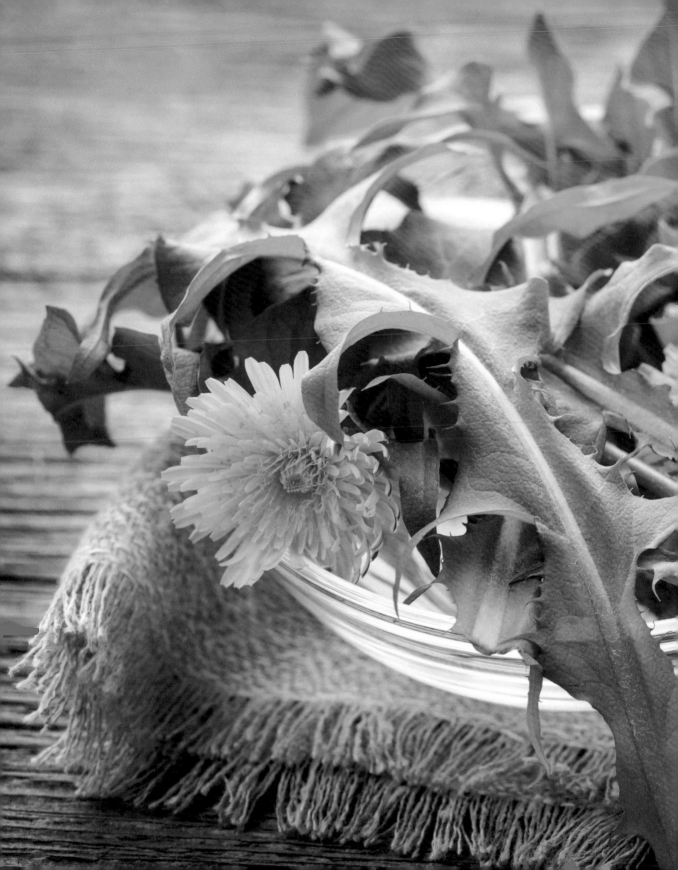

DANDELION

A wondrous "weed"

What it is: Some people think of dandelion as nothing more than a pesky weed. But the truth is, its sturdy and resilient nature means it has lots of health benefits to offer. An herbaceous perennial, dandelion (*Taraxacum officinale*) belongs to the *Asteraceae* family, along with daisies and sunflowers. It has a long history of medicinal use, particularly in traditional Chinese medicine as well as traditional Arabic, Indian, and Russian medical systems. In fact, the earliest mentions of dandelion as a therapeutic herb date back to the 10th and 11th centuries in the Middle East. All parts of the plant—roots, leaves, and flowers— can be used as medicine; the root in particular contains a wealth of health-boosting components.

What the science says: Dandelion's array of biologically active compounds, including carotenoids, sesquiterpene lactones, and chlorogenic acid, are responsible for the herb's anti-inflammatory, antioxidant, antibacterial, and antiviral properties. Research suggests dandelion may be helpful in treating urinary tract infections, as the herb exhibits antibacterial activity against the microbial offenders that most commonly cause these infections.[20] It also appears to inhibit replication of HIV and to have an antiviral effect against hepatitis B.[21, 22]

In one lab study, dandelion leaf extract was found to decrease the growth of breast cancer cells. This study also found that dandelion leaf extract blocked the invasion of prostate cancer cells, while dandelion root extract blocked the invasion of breast cancer cells (*invasion* refers to the action of cancer cells penetrating nearby tissue).[23] It's not the only study to suggest that dandelion may be a novel anticancer agent. Research demonstrates dandelion has anticancer potential in several cancer cell models, including liver, pancreatic, and colorectal cancers. What's more, the science shows it's nontoxic to healthy, noncancerous cells.

Because of its anti-inflammatory attributes, evidence is building for dandelion's ability to protect against many inflammation-driven conditions, such as atherosclerosis and other risk factors for cardiovascular disease, inflammatory bowel disease, pancreatitis, and acute lung injury.[24] And I really could go on and on. Research indicates dandelion can not only do all of the above but also reduce the risk for type 2 diabetes, help regulate blood pressure, lower the odds of obesity and help maintain a healthy weight, improve digestion, alleviate arthritis symptoms, boost bone health, promote healthy skin, and much more.

Try it: I enjoy sipping dandelion tea or juice, especially when the leaves are used in combination with aloe (see recipe on page 75). But you can also enjoy dandelion greens in meals. It's important to note that in addition to many beneficial phytochemicals, the greens are great sources of important vitamins and minerals, such as vitamins C and K and calcium. The root is also a rich source of soluble fiber. Often dandelion root is dried and ground and consumed as a coffee substitute. As a supplement, various dandelion capsules and tinctures are available.

ECHINACEA

Not just a pretty flower

What it is: One of nine herbaceous flowering plants belonging to the daisy family, echinacea—commonly called coneflower—is native to central and eastern North America. It has long been used by Native Americans to treat respiratory infections and inflammatory conditions. Early settlers took note and began using the plant as medicine themselves.

It was even listed in the *US National Formulary* of medicinal botanicals from 1916 to 1950; the publication is now called the *US Pharmacopeia and National Formulary* and shares descriptions and dosage information for both common drugs and supplements. Three species of echinacea are commonly found in herbal preparations: *Echinacea purpurea*, *Echinacea angustifolia*, and *Echinacea pallida*; their leaves, flowers, and roots can all be used. Echinacea preparations are some of the best-selling supplements in the United States and Europe.

What the science says: Science supports echinacea's general immune-stimulating properties, as well as its antiviral and antimicrobial effects. Like the other herbs discussed so far, studies in animals and humans suggest it boosts the production of important immune cells and activates critical immune processes, thus better helping these cells combat bacteria and other harmful organisms.

Studies have indeed shown benefit in regard to its use for acute upper respiratory infections like the common cold. It may shorten the duration of a cold if taken when symptoms first appear: In one placebo-controlled study of patients with colds and other upper respiratory ailments, participants with bacterial infections taking echinacea experienced illness for an average of 9.8 days, compared with 13 days in the placebo group; for viral infections, the echinacea group experienced symptoms for an average of 9.1 days versus 12.9 for the placebo group.[25]

Echinacea may also help you avoid an infection in the first place. A meta-analysis of previously published studies suggested that some preparations could reduce the risk of catching a cold by 10 to 20 percent.[26] In one trial of adults experiencing the first signs of an upper respiratory infection, 40 percent of those assigned to take echinacea progressed to a "real cold," compared with 60 percent of the placebo group. Mirroring the effects of the abovementioned study of duration, those falling ill also recovered faster, in an average of four days versus eight for those taking a placebo.[27]

Additionally, the results of one large clinical trial suggest that echinacea, at least one specific formulation of the plant, is as effective at treating the flu as a common prescription drug, and with fewer side effects to boot.[28] In the lab, echinacea has inactivated the influenza virus.[29] Early research into echinacea and cancer and other immunocompromising diseases is not conclusive, but it is promising, suggesting it may help by increasing cellular immunity.

Try it: You can find a variety of echinacea preparations, from capsules to tinctures. You can also purchase echinacea leaves in some stores and online, and the plant is easy to grow too. I use the leaves, paired with rosehips, in a healing brew (page 76).

ELDERBERRY

A bold flu fighter

What it is: The term *elderberry* refers to different varieties of plants in the genus *Sambucus*. Elderberry trees, which grow much like shrubs, produce flowers and clusters of small berries; although both have historically been regarded as medicine, it's the berries that are predominantly used in supplements today.

Black elderberry, or *Sambucus nigra*, is the most common variety and the one most typically used in herbal supplements. It's sometimes referred to as European elderberry, and its berries are a deep, rich blue-black or purple-black color. (Because of its bold hue, elderberry juice is often used as a natural colorant in food products.)

Elderberry has a long history of use for treating infections and stimulating the immune system, dating back at least to the ancient Egyptians, and it remains one of the most widely used medicinal plants in the world.

What the science says: Elderberry has demonstrated antioxidant and antimicrobial effects as well as antiviral properties, especially against the influenza virus. In fact, in the lab it has been shown to be effective against 10 different flu strains.[30] It has proved to be a flu fighter in clinical studies too.

In one randomized, placebo-controlled study of elderberry's effect on influenza subtypes A and B, 60 patients suffering from flu-like symptoms were assigned to either receive elderberry syrup or a placebo syrup four times a day for five days. On average, participants taking elderberry experienced symptom relief four days earlier than those in the placebo group, and they needed less supplemental medication than those in the placebo group as well.[31]

In another placebo-controlled study of a similar size group, participants taking elderberry experienced pronounced improvement in most flu symptoms, such as nasal congestion, fever, and muscle aches, within just 24 hours of treatment with the elderberry extract; more than half of the group experienced complete relief of their fever within 24 hours. Those in the elderberry group felt pronounced improvement in *all* flu symptoms being evaluated within 48 hours; by this time, the entire elderberry group had a complete cure of fever. Conversely, the control group experienced a worsening of symptoms over the 48-hour period.[32]

Elderberry has also been evaluated with regard to the common cold, with similar findings. In one trial among air travelers, elderberry supplementation decreased the severity of cold symptoms and the duration of illness by approximately two days.[33] Like other immune boosters, elderberry has been shown to help activate immunity by increasing production of immune cells and cytokines. It's this one–two punch that makes it so powerful: It stimulates your immune system and then targets the virus, making it even more unlikely the virus will develop resistance.

Try it: Elderberry can be found in capsules, lozenges, and gummies and as a syrup. You can also make your own syrup using dried elderberries and just a few ingredients you probably already have in your pantry; find the recipe on page 79. *Note:* Elderberries must be cooked before they can be consumed.

GARLIC

An antibacterial, anticancer allium

What it is: Yes, I'm talking about *that* garlic: The cloves sitting on your kitchen counter right now, waiting to be chopped and tossed into your next meal, are strong (pun intended) medicine. Garlic, as indicated by its scientific name, *Allium sativum*, belongs to the plant genus *Allium*; other alliums include onions, scallions, leeks, and chives. In general these species contain organosulfur compounds that offer a whole host of medicinal benefits.

They're known to be antibacterial and antimicrobial, anticarcinogenic, cardioprotective, and, of course, immune boosting—and the list goes on. Notably, garlic contains a compound called alliin. When the cloves are crushed or chewed, alliin becomes allicin. Garlic's main constituent, allicin gives it many of its medicinal properties; allicin also converts to other beneficial compounds. Although they didn't know its chemical makeup in ancient times, garlic has long been regarded as beneficial to health. Indeed, there's evidence it was so valued in ancient Egypt that it was used as currency.

What the science says: The constituents in garlic have been shown to both stimulate and suppress the immune system. In this way, garlic helps the body maintain homeostasis, or equilibrium. Specifically, garlic appears to stimulate the immune cells already discussed in these pages—macrophages, lymphocytes, natural killer cells, and dendritic cells, among others—as well as modulate the secretion of cytokines. It may also increase the production and release of nitric oxide, a molecule that acts as a defense against infectious organisms and helps regulate the growth and activity of many types of immune cells.

Garlic appears to mobilize the immune system against both bacterial and viral infections. In lab studies, it has been shown to be effective against the flu and herpes simplex viruses in particular.[34] In human research, it has also proved effective against the flu as well as the common cold. One randomized, double-blind, placebo-controlled intervention study with 120 subjects concluded that garlic (specifically aged garlic extract) reduced the severity and duration of cold and flu symptoms by 21 percent and 61 percent respectively, with researchers speculating that their findings were at least in part due to the supplement's enhancement of immune cell function.[35]

Research has shown garlic to be effective against bacteria like *Helicobacter pylori* (responsible for stomach ulcers), *E. coli* (commonly implicated in food poisoning), *Staphylococcus* (which causes staph infections), and many others. And garlic has been proven to help combat fungal infections as well.[36] Impressively, it also appears to inhibit the growth of cancer cells. Garlic's organosulfur compounds seem to block the activation, formation, and spread of carcinogenic cells. And studies suggest it may help prevent the suppression of the immune response associated with malignancy.[37]

Try it: Of course, you can enjoy fresh garlic in foods. You can also find garlic supplements in a variety of forms. One of my favorite ways to enjoy the medicinal, and not just aromatic, benefits of garlic is in a fire tonic (page 88), which also contains ginger and other beneficial ingredients. (See below to read about the powerful immune-booster ginger in its own right.)

GINGER

A spicy, medicinal powerhouse

What it is: Ginger (*Zingiber officinale*) is a flowering perennial, but it's the rhizome, or underground stem, that's widely used as a kitchen spice and a potent medicine—which is why you'll also hear it called ginger root. It belongs to the same family of plants as another herbal healer, turmeric (see page 37). Ginger has been regarded as not just a culinary but also a medicinal superstar for centuries; it was so valued in the Middle Ages that just a pound of ginger cost the same amount as one sheep. It's thought of as a traditional remedy for common problems like nausea and vomiting as well as pain. But its benefits don't end there.

What the science says: In addition to ginger's power as an analgesic and its ability to treat an array of digestive issues, research suggests it may help with degenerative disorders, heart disease, diabetes, cancer, and many other ailments. Its more than 100 biological compounds—chiefly gingerols, followed by shogaols, zingiberene, and zingerone—have been found to possess antioxidant, antimicrobial, and anti-inflammatory properties. And indeed, ginger's impact on the diseases mentioned above likely stem from its ability to tame inflammation and help keep the immune system in balance and harmony.

For instance, in one trial of patients with the autoimmune condition rheumatoid arthritis (RA), ginger supplementation was shown to significantly increase the expression of FOXP3 genes, important genes in the regulation of immune cells known as regulatory T cells. In autoimmune conditions like RA, a deficiency of T-cell activity can pave the way for other autoimmune cells to attack the body's own tissues. Conversely, the study found that ginger decreased expression of other genes that play a role in inflammation. In the end, these actions resulted in a reduced manifestation of the disease in those taking ginger.[38]

When it comes to osteoarthritis, ginger's anti-inflammatory properties have shined in studies, with research indicating it provides patients improvement in symptoms by reducing the release of pro-inflammatory cytokines from immune cells.

As for cancer, ginger may help activate the immune system to keep cancer from developing, and even to kill existing cancerous cells and keep them from spreading. It also appears to sensitize tumors to radiotherapy and chemotherapy. Studies suggest it may prove beneficial for a variety of cancers, including breast, colorectal, and prostate cancers.

Ginger's influence on inflammation and the immune system may also have a particular benefit in the management of allergic diseases such as asthma. In a novel mouse study on ginger and allergic asthma, the compound [6]-gingerol was found to suppress the immune response that triggers the condition.[39]

Try it: I always have fresh ginger root on hand to use in broth and soups (pages 93, 107, 108) and to spice up homemade chai (page 104). And I'm a big fan of ginger switchel. Not familiar? Turn to page 102 to discover this delicious drink.

GINKGO BILOBA

A hardy tree to reinforce your resilience

What it is: The ginkgo biloba tree, also called the maidenhair tree, is the oldest living tree species known to man. It's native to China, and some trees there are said to be between 2,500 and 3,000 years old (the trees typically live closer to 1,000 years). The name *ginkgo* derives from the Japanese words *gin* and *kyo*, which mean "silver" and "apricot," respectively; the ginkgo's fruit indeed resembles an apricot.

Because it's the only remaining species in the *Ginkgoaceae* family, it's sometimes referred to as a "living fossil." Ginkgo has survived, unchanged, through the Triassic, Jurassic, and Cretaceous epochs—through the time of dinosaurs roaming the land and their subsequent extinction—and even through the atomic bombing of Hiroshima. It should be no surprise, then, that the tree is known for its hardiness and resilience.

What the science says: Its resilience may also explain its powerful healing properties. Like humans, trees have immune systems. But unlike human immune systems, which begin to degenerate with age, the immune systems of 1,000-year-old ginkgo trees resemble those of 20-year-old trees. This is not to say that ginkgo is the fountain of youth (although it can help eliminate free radicals that cause wrinkles and other signs of aging), but rather that it may offer us immunological benefits, along with neuroprotective and metabolic support as well. In fact, studies suggest ginkgo is an immunostimulant with antioxidant, anti-inflammatory, and antiviral actions. Researchers believe the flavonoids in ginkgo, called ginkgolides, are primarily responsible for its widespread positive impact on health.

Studies have found ginkgo biloba extract to prevent platelets from aggregating inside arterial walls and to keep plaque from forming; it's also been found to be a vasodilator, meaning it widens blood vessels and decreases blood pressure. Thus it has important implications in preventing and treating cardiovascular disease. It may also halt the progression of dementia symptoms and protect against Alzheimer's as well, in part because of its ability to protect blood vessels and improve blood flow to the brain.

In one recent study on constituents of ginkgo called ginkgolic acids (GA), investigators reported that GA inhibits herpes simplex virus type 1 and Zika virus, as well as HIV, Ebola virus, influenza A, and Epstein–Barr

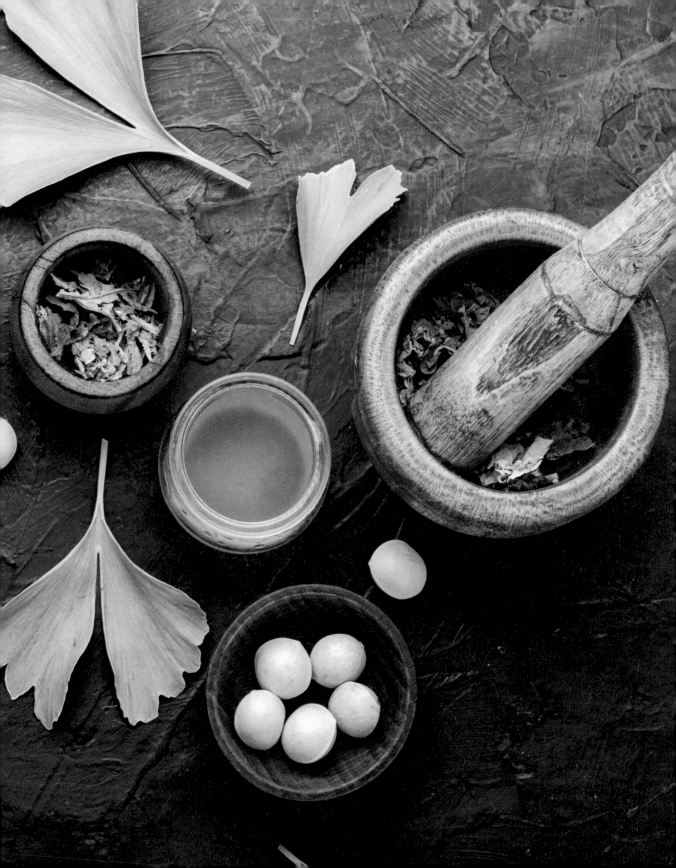

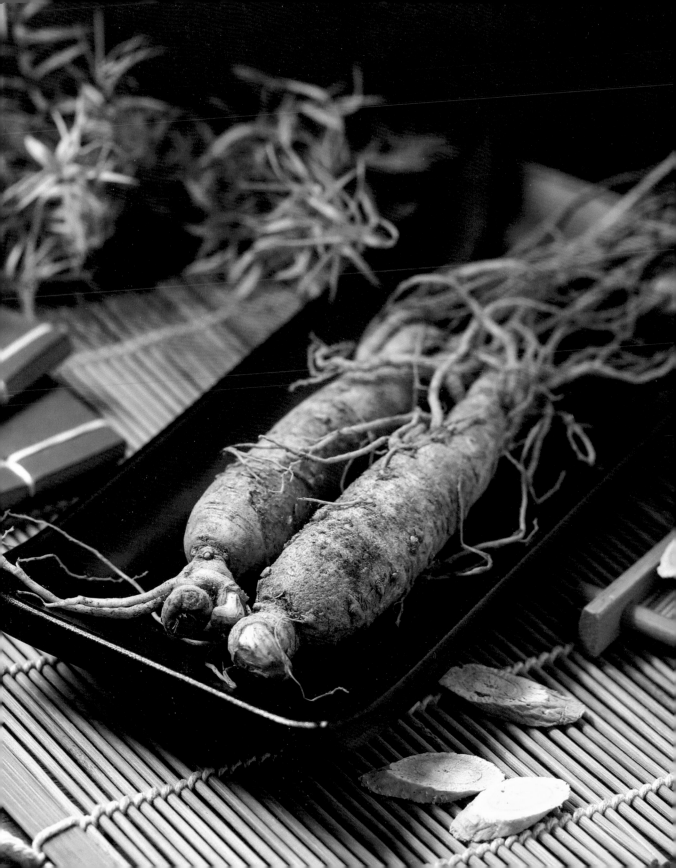

virus. Because of their impressive results, these researchers suggest ginkgo could possibly be used to treat acute viral infections, even of viruses such as coronavirus and measles.[40]

Ginkgo may also play a role in alleviating stress and anxiety. (Again, that's not surprising given the tree's ability to defend against stressors and extend its own life.) In one study, participants with generalized anxiety disorder experienced better anxiety relief after taking ginkgo than did those who took a placebo.[41]

In another, of stressed rats versus healthy controls, the immune response of stressed rats was restored after treatment with ginkgo biloba extract.[42]

Try it: Ginkgo biloba supplements are widely available in liquid extract, capsule, and tablet forms. The extract is made from the dried leaves of the plant. You can also purchase dried ginkgo leaves for use in cooking; try them in a strengthening chicken broth (page 111).

GINSENG

One of the most popular herbal supplements—and with good reason

What it is: *Ginseng* comes from a Chinese word that translates roughly to "man root." Indeed, the woody root does look a bit like a human's limbs. Ginseng has been used for some 3,000 years in traditional Chinese medicine, with many practitioners calling it the "root of longevity."

(Here, when I'm talking about ginseng, I'm referring to Asian ginseng [*Panax ginseng*] and American ginseng [*Panax quinquefolius*]. I'm *not* talking about Siberian ginseng [*Eleutherococcus senticosus*], also known as eleuthero, which isn't technically a ginseng at all.)

Ginseng is traditionally known for its ability to boost memory and energy. But its benefits don't end there. In fact, traditional herbalists categorize it as a "general tonic" able to keep the body healthy and protect it against disease, which makes good sense considering it has the capacity to stimulate the immune system. It's considered an adaptogen, like ashwagandha (page 12), which means it helps

your body withstand physical and mental stress. (Although not being discussed here, eleuthero is also an adaptogen with immune-stimulating action.)

What the science says: Ginsenosides are the main active components in ginseng—at least 36 different ginsenosides have been identified in Asian ginseng alone—responsible for the herb's immunostimulating properties as well as its antitumor and antioxidant activities. When ginsenosides function as antioxidants, they protect the outer membranes of cells, including immune cells.

Research suggests that in addition to protecting these cells' membranes, ginseng extracts also help boost immune cell activity, notably that of macrophages, T cells, and natural killer cells, thus turning on the body's anticancer defenses. In one clinical trial, 63 patients with stomach cancer were randomized to either receive chemotherapy alone or chemotherapy along with injections of an herbal combination containing ginseng.

Those who received chemotherapy and herbs experienced a significant increase in levels of T cells and natural killer cells, while those in the chemotherapy group actually showed decreases in these important immune cells. A similar result was observed in patients undergoing treatment for nasopharyngeal carcinoma who received injections of ginseng polysaccharide. Importantly, no toxic effects from the injections were reported.[43]

Studies also point to ginseng's ability to help the immune system fend off viruses and bacteria. In one randomized, placebo-controlled, double-blind trial, researchers followed participants for three months; some were given an influenza vaccine plus a placebo, while others received a flu vaccine plus a standardized ginseng extract. The group given ginseng experienced a "highly significant" reduction in incidence of upper respiratory infection (colds and flu) compared with the placebo group.

And, as with the studies mentioned above, participants who took ginseng had significantly greater natural killer cell activity—in fact, nearly twice as high as controls—at different points throughout the investigation.[44] In another study, participants given ginseng experienced fewer colds over a four-month period than did controls, as well as a reduction of cold symptoms in general and a reduction in the duration of days those cold symptoms persisted.[45]

Ginseng may also protect against a variety of bacteria, from *H. pylori* to *Staphylococcus aureus* and *E. coli*. Ginseng also appears to have antidiabetic as well as neuroprotective properties, which may make it beneficial in the treatment of Alzheimer's, Parkinson's, and other neurological disorders.

Try it: While you can take ginseng in supplement form, you can also incorporate it into your cooking. Use it to make a powerful immune-boosting broth base for a tasty seaweed and salmon soup (page 115).

GREEN TEA

Quite possibly the healthiest beverage on the planet

What it is: Like other teas, green tea is made from the leaves of the *Camellia sinensis* plant. But unlike black tea and other types, it is not oxidized. In fact, it's the least processed type of tea. (Herbal teas are not technically teas, but tisanes.) Because the leaves are only quickly heated and then dried shortly after harvest, they're abundant in polyphenol antioxidants, richer in these free-radical scavengers than other tea types.

Polyphenols can account for up to 30 percent of the dry leaf weight of green tea. In particular, green tea contains polyphenols called catechins, and specifically the powerful catechin epigallocatechin-3-gallate (EGCG), which is often isolated for studies into green tea's health benefits, and which accounts for almost 60 percent of the total polyphenol content in green tea. EGCG offers 25 to 100 times more antioxidant activity than even vitamins C and E.

What the science says: In addition to their antioxidant effects, green tea catechins, and especially EGCG, have been shown to have anti-inflammatory, antimicrobial, antiviral, antitumorigenic, and antiproliferative actions. Thus, research has found green tea to positively impact a variety of chronic diseases, including obesity, heart disease, Alzheimer's, and cancer. In general, polyphenols enhance immune function. Catechins, specifically, have been proved to maintain the activity of natural killer cells, while ECGC appears to increase regulatory T cells, which suppress autoimmunity and maintain immune tolerance.

Green tea's impact on the immune system plays a role in its well-studied antiviral activity in viruses that cause both acute and chronic infections. For instance, it has been found to inhibit the flu virus and to reduce the symptoms and duration of colds and flu. In one randomized, controlled study, participants received either a daily placebo or a green tea capsule (containing L-theanine and EGCG, equal to 10 cups of green tea) for five months. At the end of the study period, 32.1 percent fewer subjects in the green tea capsule group, relative to the placebo group, experienced cold or influenza symptoms. The green tea group also experienced 35.6 percent fewer symptom days.[46]

Studies have even found that gargling with green tea, a practice common in East Asian countries, can help prevent colds and flu.[47] Studies also report that green tea catechins may possess anti-HIV and anti-HCV activities (HCV is the hepatitis C virus, a major cause of chronic liver disease), as well as help protect against many other viruses responsible for chronic infectious diseases.[48]

A variety of different types of studies also highlight green tea's anticancer properties. Indeed, research suggests it may help reduce the risk of certain cancers, such as leukemia and cancers of the liver or lung, or may be used as an effective adjunctive treatment in bladder, breast, and colon cancers. It may also provide some protection against skin cancers caused by exposure to the sun's UV rays.[49]

Try it: While you can take green tea as a supplement (as a capsule or powder), to me, nothing is better than slowly sipping and enjoying a cup. I don't rely on bags but instead brew it myself using dried leaves along with mint; get the recipe on page 116.

LICORICE ROOT

One of the world's oldest herbal medicines

What it is: Although licorice candies are flavored with licorice root extract, they're far from medicine. But the root of the licorice plant itself, scientific name *Glycyrrhiza glabra*, has a long history as an herbal remedy. In fact, its use is documented on Assyrian clay tablets and Egyptian papyri. It was valued in ancient

Arabia for calming coughs and in ancient Greece for treating coughs and asthma. The herb has a long track record of medicinal regard in China as well, where it was used to relieve irritation of the mucous membranes and spasms in the gastrointestinal tract, as well as arthritis.

In India, Ayurvedic medicine views licorice root as an expectorant and anti-inflammatory remedy that also affects the function of the adrenal glands. Indeed, like astragalus and ginseng, it's considered an adaptogenic herb, meaning it helps your body deal with stress, by regulating the stress hormone cortisol and taking a load off your adrenals. Today, all around the world, it is still widely used in these traditional ways, especially in the management of gastrointestinal issues and respiratory infections. What's more, researchers are routinely validating these uses and uncovering new details about licorice root's pharmacological activities.

What the science says: Licorice root exhibits a broad range of properties: antibacterial, antiviral, antioxidant, anti-inflammatory, and antitumor, to name a few. Scientists have identified more than 20 triterpenoids and nearly 300 flavonoids in the licorice plant, constituents responsible for its health benefits.

Chief among these active compounds is glycyrrhizin, which is almost 50 times sweeter than sugar and demonstrates strong antiviral activity in particular. Many of the flavonoids found in licorice root have been reported to play vital roles in the proper functioning of the immune system, specifically by promoting regulatory T-cell induction, thus helping control immune response and preventing autoimmunity.

Of course, its many actions work together. Back in the late 1990s, an animal study found that licorice was effective in protecting mice exposed to a lethal amount of the influenza virus. The herb stimulated immune cell activity and the production of a cytokine critical for adaptive immunity against viral infection.[50] Since then, many studies have confirmed licorice's antiviral effect against influenza and documented its effect against herpes simplex, hepatitis, and even HIV, as well as other viruses including SARS-CoV-1, the novel coronavirus that emerged in 2003 and was known colloquially as SARS.

This suggests that glycyrrhizin could be a powerful preventive and treatment for SARS-CoV-2, the virus that causes COVID-19, which shares 79.5 percent of the SARS-CoV-1 genome's information.[51] Both of these viruses enter the cells that line the inside of human lungs through the same mechanism. A letter published in the journal *The Lancet* soon after the SARS-CoV-1 outbreak stated, "In addition to inhibition of virus replication, glycyrrhizin inhibits adsorption and penetration of the virus."[52]

NextStrain.org, which tracks viruses around the globe, has determined that the SARS-CoV-2 virus mutates 1,000 times faster than the flu virus, which means creating an effective vaccine will be 1,000 times harder than creating an effective flu vaccine. A natural compound with no known side effects that has a history of preventing the replication of a SARS-type virus, in my eyes, is a far superior avenue to pursue than a vaccine or antiviral drug that has been rushed to market with no research on possible long-term side effects.

Researchers have also delved into licorice's other properties. Studies have affirmed its use for easing congestion and making coughs more productive (loosening and expelling phlegm in viral illnesses helps reduce areas where bacteria may breed and trigger pneumonia), and it has shown antimicrobial action against *H. pylori,* the cause of many gastrointestinal ulcers. Studies have also affirmed its use in easing symptoms of acid reflux and GERD and generally improving stomach health.

As an anti-inflammatory and antioxidant, studies suggest that licorice root may be effective in treating skin issues from eczema to cysts and that it shows neuroprotective promise, with the possible ability to help prevent the degeneration that leads to dementia and Alzheimer's. Its constituents have also demonstrated antitumor activity in breast and ovarian cancer, gastric tumors, and leukemia.[53]

Try it: There is an array of licorice supplements on the market. I like to buy licorice root sticks, which I combine with other healing ingredients in a gut-soothing tea (page 127). Note that you should be careful not to overdo it with licorice. If taken in excess, the active ingredient glycyrrhiza could cause headaches, fatigue, and high blood pressure, and even heart attacks. If you want the benefits of licorice without the risks of overdosing on glycyrrhiza, deglycyrrhizinated licorice (DGL), which is licorice without glycyrrhizin, is available.

OLIVE LEAF

A remedy not to be overlooked

What it is: You've heard about the many health benefits of olive oil, which is made by grinding olives into a paste and extracting their oil. Typically the stems and leaves are discarded; some olive oil producers even charge olive farmers a fee for the disposal of the leaves. But the leaves of the olive tree (*Olea europaea*) are actually just as precious as the fruit and should be regarded not as a waste product but as powerful medicine.

Thankfully, more and more people today are realizing this. It's knowledge humans have long held, although it has been forgotten with time. In fact, the medicinal use of the leaves of the olive tree dates back thousands of years. Olive leaf is the first botanical healing herb cited in the Bible (Ezekiel 47:12): "The fruit thereof shall be for meat, and the leaf thereof for medicine." There's also recorded evidence that the ancient Egyptian and Mediterranean cultures called on the leaves to treat a variety of health conditions, including urinary tract infections, stomach issues, respiratory conditions such as asthma, and more.

What the science says: Research confirms olive leaf's medicinal benefits, demonstrating its antioxidant, anti-inflammatory, antiviral, antidiabetic, anticancer, and cardioprotective properties. It appears that the phenolic compounds present in the leaves, especially the compound oleuropein, are responsible for these attributes; the leaves contain a much higher concentration of oleuropein than the fruit.

Oleuropein has been found to be a broad-spectrum antiviral, with effect against some strains of influenza and respiratory viruses. Indeed, in one study of high school athletes, those who took a daily olive leaf extract supplement containing 100 mg of oleuropein for nine weeks during their competitive season experienced a 28 percent reduction in sick days due to upper respiratory infection compared with their peers who took a placebo.[54]

The heart benefits of oleuropein were first noted back in the 1950s, when it was found to have hypotensive action and to dilate blood vessels. Studies have since found it may also play a role in preventing cardiovascular diseases by limiting the formation of arterial plaque through inhibiting LDL oxidation. And research has shown that olive leaf extracts may possess antispasmodic, vasodilator, and antiarrhythmic properties.

Olive leaf's many positive impacts on health are due at least in part to its ability to act as a modulator of the human immune response. Research suggests it increases levels of nitric oxide, said to be one of the most versatile players in the immune system, involved in the control of infectious and chronic diseases, autoimmunity, and tumors. Studies also indicate that it boosts numbers of natural killer cells and maintains a balance between regulatory T cells and other immune cells.

Researchers responsible for these findings link olive leaf's immune-modulating properties to its cardioprotective effects and ability to prevent cardiovascular events, as well as to its potential therapeutic use in the treatment of chronic inflammatory disease and its anti-tumor activity.[55] Other research indicates that olive leaf extract may kill cancer cells as well as inhibit the proliferation of cancerous cells.

Try it: You can find olive leaf as a powder, extract, or tablet, or you can purchase the dried leaves themselves. That's what I like to do: I combine dried olive leaf and dried lemon balm leaf in a healing tea; see page 128.

OREGANO

Much more than a pizza spice

What it is: There are reportedly at least 60 species and 17 genera, belonging to several different botanical families, called "oregano." The herb most people know as oregano, *Origanum vulgare*, belongs to the mint family (*Lamiaceae*); you may hear it referred to as Greek oregano or wild marjoram. The word *oregano* stems from ancient Greek and translates to "mountain joy," and indeed, the ancient Greeks and Romans revered it as a symbol of happiness: Drawings from the time show brides and grooms wearing crowns of oregano leaves. The plant has a long history of use as both a culinary seasoning and a medicine. Traditional medicinal uses have included treating colds and other respiratory infections as well as digestive disorders.

What the science says: Oregano contains a number of interesting phytonutrients that help give it a well-deserved reputation for healing. Specifically, it's abundant in flavonoids and phenolic acids, especially rosmarinic acid and thymol, dietary consumption of which has been associated with a decreased risk of chronic disease. In fact, these constituents appear to be powerful antioxidant, anti-inflammatory, and anticancer agents.

As you know, antioxidants lower oxidative stress in the body caused by free radicals and thus strengthen the immune system. Not only have herbs in general been found to have higher antioxidant activity than fruits and vegetables, but oregano appears to rank highest in this regard. In one study of 39 commonly used herbs, all grown in the same location and under the same conditions, oregano was found to deliver up to 20 times more antioxidant activity than the other herbs studied.[56]

Of course, antioxidants also help prevent the free radical damage that is associated with cancer. One review of previously published studies found that extracts from different species of oregano were toxic to a variety of human cancer cells, including breast, lung, and central nervous system cancer cells. They have also been shown to inhibit the growth and spread of breast, liver, and colorectal cancer cells.[57]

Research into oregano's impact on breast cancer in particular is ongoing—and promising. In one recent animal study, even low doses of freeze-dried oregano suppressed the frequency of breast tumors by more than 55 percent, as well as suppressed tumor volume and incidence, when compared with control animals. High-dose oregano supplementation lengthened the period of tumor dormancy by 12.5 days. In both high- and low-dose animal groups, oregano decreased the viability and proliferation of cancerous cells. On the basis of their findings, the researchers were able to say, "Our results demonstrate, for the first time, a distinct tumor-suppressive effect of oregano in the breast cancer model."[58]

And its benefits don't end there: Oregano is also abundant in the compound carvacrol, which has been found to possess antibacterial, antifungal, and liver- and blood-vessel-protective properties, as well as antioxidant, anticancer, and anti-inflammatory attributes.[59] In addition to the specific conditions mentioned already, oregano may prove helpful with everything from allergies and headaches to acne and tooth pain.

Try it: There are countless ways to incorporate oregano into your meals. I use it to flavor many dishes, including Steak with Oregano and Roasted Garlic Sauce (page 131). You'll even find it in my Fire Tonic (page 88). You may also consider having essential oil of oregano around to use topically and on surfaces as an antimicrobial.

REISHI

A miraculous mushroom

What it is: Reishi (*Ganoderma lucidum*), also known as lingzhi, has been called the "mushroom of immortality"—and for good reason, as you'll come to find out. The glossy, dark-reddish, kidney-shaped mushroom grows at the base of deciduous trees and has been used medicinally, even worshiped as an herbal remedy, in Asian countries for thousands of years. Its medicinal value was written about in a 2,000-year-old Chinese medical text, and it's reported that Chinese and Japanese emperors regularly drank mushroom teas and concoctions containing reishi for vitality and longevity. They were certainly on to something.

What the science says: The reishi mushroom has been found to contain roughly 400 different biologically active compounds with a vast array of pharmacological effects—so many, in fact, that I'm hard pressed to list them all here. Reishi and its constituents have demonstrated immune-modulating, anti-atherosclerotic, analgesic, anti-inflammatory, antitumor, antibacterial, antiviral, antiparasitic, antifungal, antioxidant, hypotensive and hypertensive, antiallergic, cardioprotective, and hypoglycemic properties—and there are many more I could name. Scientific results have been so impressive that reishi is now recognized as an adjuvant, or complement, in diabetes, hepatitis, carcinoma, and leukemia treatments.

To be sure, its widespread health benefits are in large part due to its immune-modulating actions and ability to enhance and support immune function. Reishi constituents, such as the triterpene ganoderic acid, have been found to activate many of the immune cells already mentioned, such as macrophages, natural killer cells, T lymphocytes, and B cells. This activation then leads to the production of various cytokines and anti-inflammatory and other effects.[60]

These cells are important in the fight against cancer. For example, natural killer cells are specific types of white blood cells with powerfully destructive capabilities against tumors; T lymphocytes also seek and destroy pathogens and may help combat cancer. As mentioned above, reishi is currently being used to help treat carcinoma, especially lung carcinoma. And indeed, research has found ganoderic acid from reishi to destroy human lung carcinoma cell lines and to suppress tumor growth and proliferation.[61] It has also demonstrated the same effects in inflammatory breast cancer cells.[62]

Reishi's constituents also inhibit the release of histamine from mast cells. The presence of histamine initiates the allergic response, when the immune system treats normally harmless substances in the environment as harmful; thus, research has found the mushroom to be useful in managing allergies. Reishi restores the balance between immune states that are out of whack in people with allergies. That's exciting because allergies are increasing in frequency, and because traditional medicines treat only their symptoms. Because reishi balances the immune system's response, it treats the underlying cause of allergies.[63]

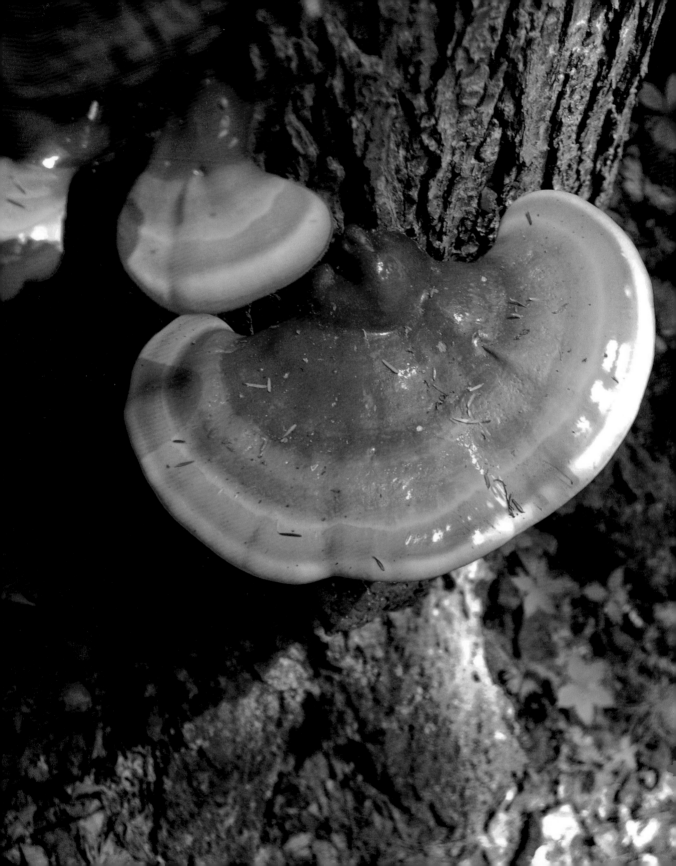

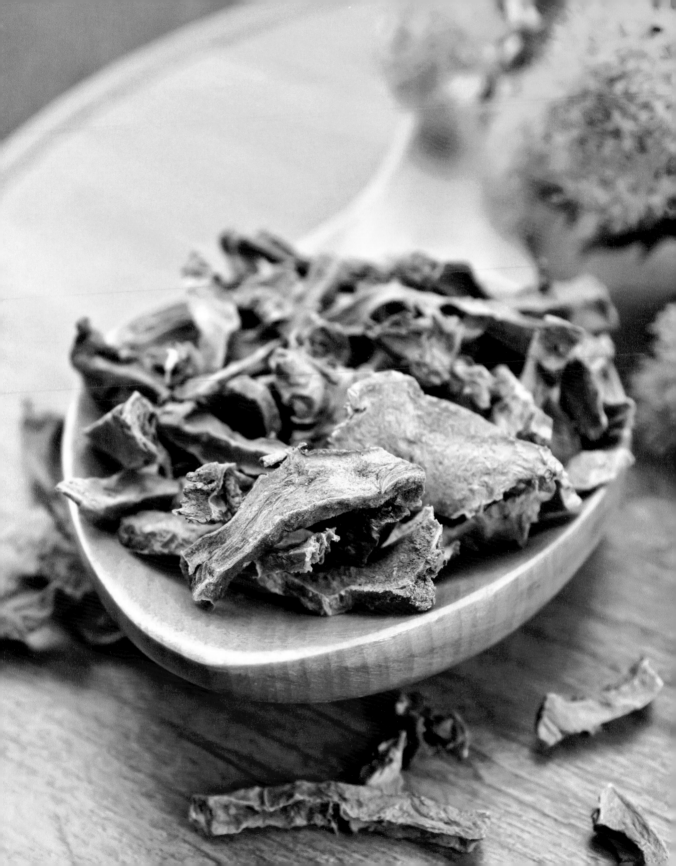

Try it: Find dried reishi slices and powder for cooking, as well as supplements in capsule form. I like to use the powder, to do as ancient emperors did and make a delicious drink. There are many other wonderfully healing mushrooms out there, including turkey tail (page 36), so feel free to use a blend of mushroom powders in my Mushroom Latte recipe on page 133.

RHODIOLA

A hardy healer

What it is: *Rhodiola rosea* is a tough perennial, typically found in the arctic areas of Europe and Asia, that produces beautiful, chrysanthemum-like flowers. Its red, pink, or yellow blooms are quite fragrant when cut, so they're sometimes used as a substitute for roses. In fact, it's often called rose root, as well as golden root and king's crown. But rhodiola has a lot more going for it than its attractive appearance and scent. For millennia, people familiar with the plant have used it to improve strength and virility.

For instance, Siberian brides were given rhodiola sprigs to boost their physical endurance to face long, subzero winters, as well as to increase fertility and fend off anxiety and depression. Indeed, rhodiola is an adaptogenic herb, like ginseng (page 25), meaning it helps the body adapt to stress—and we know chronic stress can weaken the immune system. It has long been a mainstay of the traditional medicines of Sweden, Norway, Iceland, and Russia and was even written about in a renowned ancient Greek medical text dating all the way back to sometime around the year 70 C.E.

What the science says: This adaptogenic herb contains more than 140 powerful compounds responsible for its benefits to health, notably tyrosol and salidroside (rhodioloside), the latter of which is considered by many to be the plant's most important bioactive molecule. These constituents have been found to have, in addition to adaptogenic properties, antifatigue, antidepressant, antioxidant, anti-inflammatory, anticancer, antiviral, and, not surprisingly, immune-modulating activities. Among other actions, it appears to stimulate and protect the immune system by normalizing hormones and regulating the glucocorticoid levels in the body, as well as by decreasing levels of certain inflammatory cytokines secreted by immune cells. It has also been found to bolster important immune T cells.

Rhodiola has been shown to protect athletes from viral infections. In one study, 48 marathon runners randomly received either 600 mg of rhodiola or a placebo for four weeks prior to a race. Blood samples were collected at three intervals: before the start of the race, and 15 minutes and 90 minutes after the race's end. Follow-up using in vitro assays indicated that rhodiola was able to protect cells against the vesicular stomatitis virus for 12 hours after physical exertion.[64]

Research looking into rhodiola's anticancer activity is also promising. In cell culture studies, rhodiola has been found to inhibit cell proliferation and induce cell death in a variety of cancers, including bladder, breast, colorectal, stomach, and lung cancers. Anecdotal evidence from one clinical study suggested that when patients with superficial bladder carcinoma were given rhodiola, the average frequency of relapses was reduced by half.[65]

Try it: Rhodiola supplements are widely available, and rhodiola tea can be found in health food stores, tea shops, and online. Find out how I brew up a cup on page 134.

TURKEY TAIL

A mushroom catching the eye of foragers and scientists alike

What it is: Turkey tail mushroom (*Trametes versicolor*, also known as *Coriolus versicolor*) is so called because it resembles a wild turkey's tail in both shape and color. Its flesh has a leathery texture and appears rust brown or orange in areas, dark brown or blackish in some spots, and light brown or whitish in others. You may also hear this fungus called a cloud mushroom. It's long been used in traditional Chinese medicine to boost the immune system, and in particular to combat cancer. And the science is now confirming what traditional Chinese medicine practitioners have long known: Turkey tail is a powerful immune system enhancer that holds an arsenal of cancer-blasting compounds.

What the science says: Medicinal mushrooms like turkey tail and reishi (see page 32) support the immune system in a variety of ways. Turkey tail specifically has been found to enhance the innate and adaptive immune responses: It increases the production of immune-activating cytokines and antiviral cytokines and also boosts the production of markers that are part of regenerative processes involving stem cells.[66]

Constituents called polysaccharides are thought to be generally responsible for medicinal mushrooms' immunological effects. Two specific polysaccharide complexes in turkey tail—the proteoglycans polysaccharide peptide (PSP) and polysaccharide-K (PSK, or Krestin)—are getting a great deal of scientific attention, including large-scale clinical trials. Thanks to these compounds, turkey tail has become the most extensively researched of all the medicinal mushrooms out there.

In one major clinical study funded by the National Institutes of Health, turkey tail was found to improve immune function in women with stage I, II, or III breast cancer. The increase in immune cell counts and activity in participants was dose-dependent, meaning the higher the dose of turkey tail preparation they received, the greater the boost in immune response they experienced. What's more, no serious adverse events from the turkey tail were reported.[67]

Turkey tail has been found to hold immense promise for several other cancers as well. PSP in particular has been shown to significantly enhance immune status in 70 to 97 percent of patients with stomach, esophageal, lung, ovarian, and cervical cancers.[68] In another study, PSK was found to be effective against stage II and III colon cancer: The researchers found that patients given a derivative from turkey tail had an 86.8 percent survival rate, compared with a 60 percent survival rate in the control group.

Turkey tail is also being used to treat many different bacterial, fungal, and viral infections, including *Aspergillus niger*, *Candida albicans*, *E. coli*, HIV, herpes, and streptococcus pneumonia; it is also hepatoprotective and may prevent liver damage.

Try it: Find turkey tail in capsules, as a powder, and as a liquid extract. I use the powder to create a tea, typically combining it with reishi and other medicinal mushrooms (page 133).

TURMERIC

A golden remedy

What it is: Turmeric is a bold herb in every sense of the word. It's responsible for mustard's distinct yellow hue, and it lends a brilliant color as well as a warm, peppery flavor to Indian curry dishes. From the rhizome, or underground stem, of the *Curcuma longa* plant, turmeric root has orange flesh and an earthy scent more pungent than ginger. The plant actually belongs to the ginger family, and the two relatives are often used together medicinally. Because of its numerous health benefits, turmeric has earned the nickname "the spice of life"; you may also hear it called "Indian saffron." It has a long history of use in Ayurvedic and traditional Chinese medicine, and research confirms its benefits in a wide array of conditions that affect nearly every bodily system.

What the science says: Curcumin is arguably the most important, and most studied, active ingredient in turmeric—you may even hear or see turmeric referred to simply as curcumin.

This compound alone has been estimated to confer some 150 different therapeutic benefits. Indeed, lab and clinical data demonstrate its effectiveness in helping prevent and treat everything from cancer to cardiovascular, neurologic, metabolic, skin, and inflammatory diseases. In fact, it's been proved so effective as an anti-inflammatory that it has been compared to powerful prescription medications, but without the side effects. It makes sense, then, that it would be so potent against disease, as inflammation is involved in nearly every chronic condition we know of.

Turmeric actually battles inflammation at the molecular level. The transcription factor nuclear factor kappa-B (NF-kB) passes into a cell's nucleus, where it can "switch on" the genes related to inflammation in a number of serious chronic diseases. But curcumin is able to prevent NF-kB from turning on those inflammatory genes. What's more, curcumin also inhibits the expression of pro-inflammatory enzymes and cytokines. In this regard it's been found to be helpful in treating inflammatory bowel diseases and the joint pain and swelling of arthritis, among many other inflammatory conditions. Curcumin's capacity to modulate the immune system stems from its impact on the molecular components involved in the inflammatory process, as well as its interactions with various immune cells.[69]

A great deal of research in recent years has been dedicated to curcumin's neuroprotective properties, and especially to its potential role in treating Alzheimer's disease. Findings suggest that curcumin binds to beta-amyloid molecules and tau proteins—a buildup of which occurs in Alzheimer's and leads to the damage of brain cells essential for learning and memory—thereby helping to prevent neurodegeneration.[70]

Other recent studies have evaluated curcumin as an anticancer agent. It's been found to inhibit the growth of gastrointestinal and liver cancers as well as head and neck tumors, and to be able to target breast cancer cells.[71] In one notable study, men with colon lesions, which can turn cancerous, were given 4 grams of curcumin a day for 30 days. At the end of the study, they had a significant 40 percent reduction in the number of lesions.[72]

Not to sound like a broken record, but curcumin has been found to have a therapeutic effect on numerous diseases affecting numerous major body systems, and it really is impossible to list them all here. Suffice to say, turmeric is truly solid gold.

Try it: My favorite way to use turmeric in cooking is in delicious drinks and savory, rich broths, incorporating both the fresh root and the ground powder. Find recipes featuring turmeric beginning on page 138.

THE IMPORTANCE OF VITAMINS

In the previous section on herbs and spices, I talked about the different types of immune-boosting phytonutrients they contain, many of which you may not have heard of before, such as flavonoids, curcumin, and apigenin. But the letter vitamins you've been learning about since you were a child are just as important to promoting and maintaining immunity.

A vital immune system depends on a balanced intake of vitamins and minerals, along with lifestyle choices like exercise and sleep. It's ideal to obtain your vitamins and minerals from the foods you eat (whole and organic choices, as well as locally grown and in-season options) rather than from supplements, whenever possible.

It has always been my belief and teaching that supplements should be taken in addition to—and not in place of—a good, sound diet. You can't cover your nutrition or lifestyle "sins" by taking a handful of supplements; biology simply doesn't work that way. The most powerful tool you have to achieve good health is eating the highest-quality toxin-free foods you can find.

That's because when you obtain your vitamins from food, you also get a broad spectrum of accessory micronutrients that are vital for wellness, such as trace minerals and other supporting dietary components. They all work synergistically, in concert with one another, helping to ensure proper nutrient absorption at proper levels. This prevents you from getting too much of anything and tipping the balance in your body too far in one direction. That's the wisdom of nature.

What's more, supplements often contain synthetic versions of these nutrients. These nonnatural alternatives aren't easily absorbed by your body and may not function as well as their natural equivalents. Additionally, depending on their quality, they may come with unwanted side effects, often due to the additives they contain. For example, research has shown that the flowing agent magnesium stearate actually suppresses the natural killer cells that are a key component of your immune system.[1]

Let's look at the 13 vitamins' specific impacts on immunity and the food sources highest in them. Note that while many studies mentioned below illustrating these vitamins' benefits involve supplementation, that's usually in cases of severe deficiency and for controlled research purposes. It's still ideal to get your vitamins from your foods for optimal health and well-being. After we look at vitamins, I'll discuss two of the most important antioxidant minerals to incorporate into your diet as well.

VITAMIN A

Vitamin A boosts immunity, lowers the risk of infection, and supports wound healing by building collagen strength. Indeed, the science suggests that vitamin A deficiency is involved in many infectious diseases and that supplementation in those who are deficient may play a role in the treatment of these ailments.

For example, a cohort study on tuberculosis found that vitamin A deficiency is associated with tuberculosis occurrence, and a lab study found that retinoic acid, a form of vitamin A, inhibits the growth and survival rate of tuberculosis bacteria. Vitamin A has also demonstrated a therapeutic effect on respiratory infections and contagious diseases in children, such as pneumonia; measles; and hand, foot, and mouth disease.[2]

Foods rich in vitamin A include:

- Liver from grass-fed or pastured animals
- Wild-caught Alaskan salmon
- Organic eggs from pastured chickens

Foods rich in beta carotene, precursor to vitamin A, include:

- Squash
- Sweet potatoes
- Dark leafy greens*
- Cantaloupe

* Note: Dark leafy greens such as spinach and chard are also abundant in oxalates, or oxalic acid. While not harmful in and of itself, an overaccumulation of oxalates can trigger the development of kidney stones and may even lead to urinary tract problems, mitochondrial dysfunction, and other issues. Eating high-oxalate foods in combination with a calcium-rich food, such as butter or sour cream, will mitigate some of the harm by allowing calcium to bind to some oxalates in your intestine, thereby decreasing the risk of kidney stone formation. Still, while it's important to incorporate these vegetables into your diet for vitamins and other nutrients, you may want to do so in moderation. Also, if you have a damaged gut lining, it will increase your absorption of oxalates; in this case, you may want to get your vitamin A and other vitamins from different food sources.

VITAMIN D

Vitamin D can modulate both the innate (natural or native) and adaptive (acquired) immune responses. A deficiency in vitamin D is associated with autoimmunity: Epidemiological evidence links it to disorders from multiple sclerosis to lupus to inflammatory bowel disease. Deficiency has also been linked to increased susceptibility to infection, while supplementation has been linked to decreased risk. For instance, in one double-blind placebo study, those taking vitamin D versus placebo experienced a 42 percent lower incidence of flu infection.[3]

It's important to get regular, sensible sun exposure to optimize your vitamin D levels. While duration will vary depending on the darkness of your skin, in general this means 20 minutes a day of sun exposure on as much of the skin of your body as you can expose. If your skin is very fair, it may take some time for you to be able to be in the sun for 20 minutes without getting a sunburn (something you always want to avoid). In that case, stay in the sun until your skin just begins to turn pink. Vitamin A and vitamin D work together synergistically (along with vitamin K2; see below), and one of the easiest ways to ensure an appropriate and beneficial ratio between the two is to get the majority of your vitamin D from the sun and your vitamin A from clean animal proteins such as those listed above. However, there are times you may need to turn to your diet for vitamin D, particularly if you work primarily indoors or otherwise can't get regular sun exposure.

Foods that offer up vitamin D:

- Liver from grass-fed or pastured animals
- Wild-caught Alaskan salmon
- Organic eggs from pastured chickens

VITAMIN C

Like vitamin D, vitamin C supports both your innate and your adaptive immunity. It also acts as an antioxidant within your cells, helping to protect immune cells from damage. And it may promote the production of interferon, which helps defend against viruses. Research suggests vitamin C can help ameliorate the incidence, severity, and duration of respiratory infections including the common cold, and that it may have a beneficial effect on pneumonia recovery as well.[4]

Some of the most vitamin C–rich foods include:

- Citrus fruits
- Dark leafy greens (see note on page 40)
- Bell peppers
- Broccoli
- Berries

VITAMINS K1 AND K2

Vitamin K1 is important for healthy blood clotting, and vitamin K2 plays a major role in bone health. In general, vitamin K also affects immune and inflammatory responses, and studies have found links between vitamin K levels and inflammatory diseases.

In the lab, vitamin K2 has been found to inhibit the production of pro-inflammatory molecules by immune cells.[5] Note that the effect of vitamin D is dependent on the presence of vitamin K, and that vitamin D deficiency is actually caused by vitamin K2 deficiency. Again, this is why it's important to get your vitamins from whole foods, where they're already in balance thanks to the wisdom of nature.

Look to these foods:

- Dark leafy greens (for K1; see note on page 40)
- Animal foods (for K2)
- Fermented foods like sauerkraut; brined, unpasteurized pickles; and kimchi (for K2)

B VITAMINS

Each B vitamin—B1 (thiamine), B2 (riboflavin), B3 (niacin), B5 (pantothenic acid), B6 (pyridoxine), B7 (biotin), B9 (folate), and B12 (cobalamin)—is important for different reasons. But generally speaking, "B" is for boosting your immunity. These vitamins are especially effective when you combine the foods that contain them so they can all work together for maximum benefit.

B12 in particular is a powerful cold and flu fighter, while B9 helps repair tissues and aids in immune support and B6 naturally benefits and strengthens your immune system. In one study, vitamin B6 injections increased the immune response in critically ill subjects, boosting their numbers of important immune cells like lymphocytes and T-suppressor cells.[6]

Good dietary sources of B vitamins include:

- Dark leafy greens (see note on page 40)
- Wild-caught Alaskan salmon
- Pastured, organic chicken
- Nutritional yeast
- Raw, organic milk, yogurt, and cheese from grass-fed animals

CONSUME ANTIOXIDANT- AND MINERAL-RICH FOODS

As I've already emphasized, a vital immune system depends on a balanced intake of vitamins and minerals through a healthy diet—along with careful supplementation when appropriate and necessary. Now I'm going to focus on two essential minerals in particular that act as antioxidants in the body: zinc and selenium. These nutrients are powerful immune boosters that are easy to obtain from delicious whole foods.

ZINC

Zinc is the second most abundant trace mineral in your body, and it plays a key role in many biological processes, from thyroid function to the senses of smell and taste. Zinc is sometimes called a gatekeeper of immune function, and it's true that your entire immune system depends on this mineral to work as it should to keep you well.

The production and activity of numerous important immune cells are dependent on zinc; these include cytokines, the immune system's main messengers. Zinc also helps create and activate your immune system's white blood cells and is essential in the enzymatic reactions needed for wound healing.

As a potent antioxidant, zinc also protects against oxidative stress and assists with DNA repair. Oxidative stress occurs when there's an overabundance of free radicals. High levels of oxidative stress affect every organ and system in your body and are thus linked to all kinds of conditions, including Alzheimer's and cancer. Antioxidants counteract or neutralize the harmful effects of free radicals, so the more antioxidants you consume, the more likely your body will be able to fight back and stay healthy. Zinc also possesses anti-inflammatory properties.

Given this information, it's no surprise that zinc deficiency is implicated in multiple chronic diseases, including those associated with inflammation and oxidative stress, such as diabetes, rheumatoid arthritis, dementia, and atherosclerosis. That these are primarily diseases of aging is also no coincidence: Estimates vary, but according to some researchers, upwards of 40 percent of the American elderly population may be zinc deficient.

Alcoholics, vegetarians, women who are pregnant or lactating, and individuals who have a digestive disorder or sickle cell disease are more likely to have a zinc deficiency. Even if you consider yourself to be a healthy person, you may not be eating enough zinc-rich foods on a daily basis to achieve optimal levels of this essential nutrient. That's because, perhaps surprisingly, your body does not store zinc; instead, zinc has to be consumed, either through foods or a supplement, every day.

What are optimal levels? According to the Food and Nutrition Board of the Institute of Medicine, the recommended daily allowance (RDA) to meet the nutrient requirements for most people age 19 and older, is as follows:

- Men: 11 mg
- Women: 8 mg
- In pregnancy: 11 mg
- During lactation: 12 mg

What are good food sources? Fortunately, a wide variety of foods contain zinc, especially grass-fed red meat; pastured, organic poultry; and nuts and seeds. Oysters are actually the richest food source of zinc. You can also get zinc from hemp and sesame seeds, dairy products like yogurt and cheddar cheese, and other seafood choices.

Here are some of these foods I recommend, as well as their zinc content, to help give you a good idea of how easily, with just a little focus and planning, you can meet these values through your diet.

- Beef, lean chuck roast, 3 ounces = 7 mg (aim for 5 to 7 ounces of grass-fed red meat per day)
- Ground beef, lean, 3 ounces = 5.3 mg (aim for 5 to 7 ounces of grass-fed red meat per day)
- Pork loin, lean, 3 ounces = 2.9 mg
- Chicken, dark meat, 3 ounces = 2.4 mg

What do studies show? Because of its ability to bolster the immune system, zinc has been found to help shorten the duration of the common cold by an average of 33 percent. An analysis of previously published studies found that, depending on the type of zinc used, the length of colds were shortened by 28 to 40 percent, with similar effects found for both low and high doses.[1]

Zinc has also been found to be effective in reducing the severity of the common cold, especially when started within 24 hours of experiencing symptoms.[2] Excitingly, in combination with a zinc ionophore (zinc transport molecule), zinc has also been shown to inhibit the SARS coronavirus in vitro. In cell culture, it blocked viral replication within minutes.[3]

SELENIUM

Not only does selenium play a role in the absorption and bioavailability of zinc, but it's also an essential mineral of vital importance to health all on its own, with antioxidant, anti-inflammatory, antiviral, and anticancer properties. At the cellular level, selenium is an active component of the enzyme glutathione peroxidase. This enzyme has potent antioxidant properties and serves as a first line of defense against the buildup of harmful free radicals in your cells. Because one of the reasons people develop cancer is excessive free radical production, which you'll read more about in a minute, selenium helps reduce your risk of cancer.

Selenium also has the potential to influence the immune response via selenoproteins (selenium-containing proteins); adequate levels of the mineral help initiate immunity as well as regulate excessive immune response and chronic inflammation. Animal research has shown a selenium deficiency to result in poorer immune responses to viruses, tumors, and allergens, relative to a group with adequate selenium levels.[4]

What are optimal levels? Though selenium is absolutely critical to health, you need only a little bit of this mineral to keep your immune system and other functions humming along properly. In fact, it's considered a micronutrient and is measured in micrograms (mcg).

The U.S. RDA for those 19 years and older is as follows:

- Men and women: 55 mcg
- In pregnancy: 60 mcg
- During lactation: 70 mcg

The World Health Organization recommends higher levels, and I tend to agree. However, I do suggest that you moderate your selenium intake, because too much is associated with an increased risk of high cholesterol and diabetes, and I believe you should not exceed 200 mcg of selenium a day. You're not likely to overdose on it from the foods you eat, but you could get too much from selenium supplements. You may have low levels of selenium if you smoke cigarettes, drink alcohol, have had weight-loss surgery, or have Crohn's disease or ulcerative colitis.

What are good food sources? Brazil nuts and organic, grass-fed beef, turkey, and chicken are great sources of selenium, as are some fish (like wild-caught Alaskan salmon) and mushrooms. In fact, Brazil nuts average 70 to 90 mcg of selenium *per nut*, meaning that eating just a few a day will get you the appropriate intake of this mineral. To compare, 3 ounces of turkey contains 31 mcg of selenium, while the same amount of chicken contains around 22 mcg and ground beef around 18 mcg.

What do the studies say? As mentioned above, selenium's antioxidant protection and immune-enhancing effects mean it has anticancer properties. And indeed, research suggests high selenium levels are linked with a decrease in the risk of colorectal, prostate, and lung cancers, with a 50 to 63 percent lower incidence of these cancers; the greatest impact was seen for prostate cancer.

Selenium may also be beneficial in inhibiting HIV. Low levels of the mineral have been associated with greater progression of the disease and higher related mortality, while supplementation with selenium has correlated with slower progression and improved immune cell counts.[5] Research also suggests selenium may help combat other viral infections, like the flu, as well as bacterial infections, and may even help those with allergies and asthma.

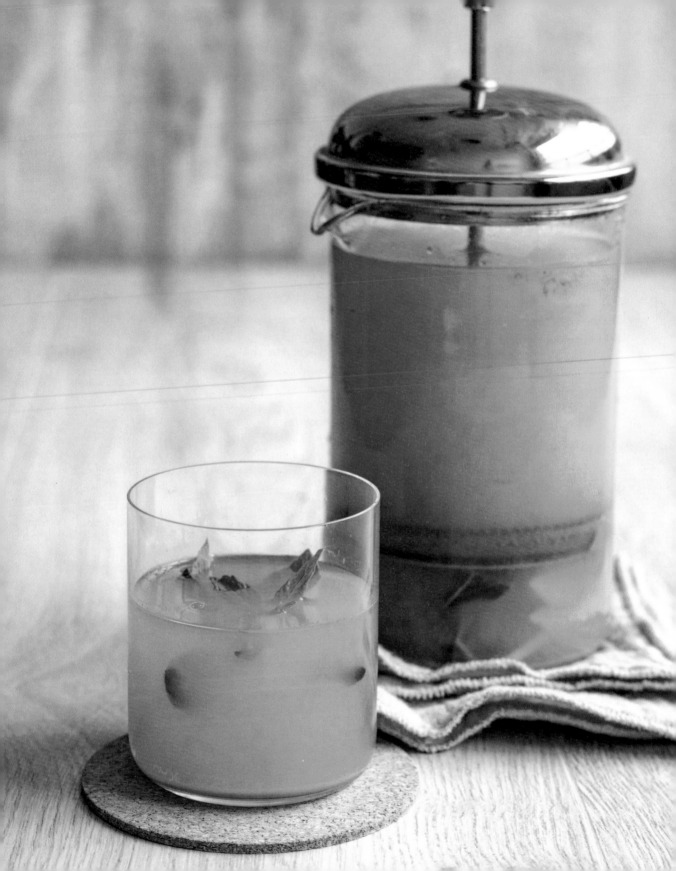

OPTIMIZE GUT HEALTH

You may have heard the statistic that about 80 percent of your immune system resides in your gut. It's true: Your body, and especially your gut, is colonized by trillions of microbes, collectively called the microbiome. These bacteria and other microorganisms, often referred to as beneficial or friendly bacteria, play a major role in immunity.

In fact, your gut microbiome regulates immune homeostasis: It keeps your immune system strong and able to defend against invading pathogens, but not so strong that it becomes overactive and shifts toward auto-immunity, attacking your own healthy tissues. Your gut is also home to a vibrant community of immune cells that defend against disease, and new research suggests these cells and gut microorganisms may interact with one another to maintain health.[1] It's fascinating, and emerging, stuff.

We know about the connection between the gut microbiome and immunity in particular largely thanks to animal research, specifically studies in germ-free mice that are born without any colonizing bacteria at all. These animals have undeveloped immune systems that lack vital immune cells. But when they are provided with beneficial bacteria, scientists have seen that their immune systems become more mature and developed.

Over the years, a wide array of animal and human studies have further shed light on the strong link between gut health and immune health. Research has clearly shown that when your gut microbiome is out of whack in any way—because of a poor diet high in processed foods, antibiotics and other drugs, or even the use of antibacterial products—your immune system gets out of balance too. This can potentially result in not only gastrointestinal diseases like inflammatory bowel disease but also other chronic conditions, including autoimmune disorders such as rheumatoid arthritis, as well as neurodegenerative diseases and cancer.[2]

On the flip side, when things are right in your gut, your body can resist autoimmunity and these conditions—even malignancy. In a recent mouse study, one type of beneficial gut bacterium was shown to reduce the number and size of colon tumors and the amount of pro-inflammatory, cancer-associated molecules in the blood. This suggests that friendly gut microbiota may not only help prevent serious diseases like cancer but also help to treat them.[3] So, how can you maintain optimal intestinal flora, so that your gut can help you sustain optimal overall health and well-being? Focus on fiber and pump up your intake of probiotic-rich foods, adding supplements when needed.

Focus on Fiber

Fiber helps balance your gut microbiome and improve your immune system, as digestion-resistant starches act as prebiotics to feed the healthy bacteria in your gut. What's more, fiber promotes bowel movements and keeps waste progressing smoothly through your colon, while at the same time benefiting your heart health and controlling your blood sugar.

There are two types of fiber: soluble, which easily dissolves in water and becomes gel-like, and insoluble, which doesn't dissolve but stays basically intact as it moves through your colon. Both types are important for digestion and overall health. National fiber recommendations call for a fiber intake of 30 to 38 grams a day for men, and 21 to 25 grams a day for women. However, my recommendation for an ideal fiber intake stands at 50 grams per 1,000 calories consumed, usually from fiber-rich foods.

To significantly raise your fiber intake, try incorporating these 10 notable fiber-rich choices:

- **Split peas and green peas**—Despite their small size, peas are a very good fiber source. Cooked split peas contain roughly 16.3 grams of fiber per cup, while cooked green peas have 8.8 grams of fiber per cup.
- **Artichokes**—Fiber is one of the main nutrients in artichokes. A medium-size cooked artichoke delivers about 10 grams of fiber.
- **Raspberries**—A cup of these sweet antioxidant-rich berries has 8 grams of fiber.
- **Collard greens**—These low-calorie leafy greens contain around 7.6 grams of fiber per cup. (See my note on page 40 about greens.)
- **Blackberries**—These berries contains both soluble and insoluble fiber; a cup has 7.6 grams of this nutrient.
- **Avocados**—Avocados aren't just a source of healthy fats that are vital for overall health. Half an avocado typically contains 6.7 grams of fiber.
- **Pears**—A medium-size pear has 5.5 grams of fiber, alongside phytonutrients like beta-carotene, lutein, and zeaxanthin.
- **Spinach**—Spinach is another fiber-rich leafy green; just 1 cup provides about 4 grams of fiber. (See my note on page 40 about greens.)
- **Brussels sprouts**—One cup of boiled brussels sprouts can deliver around 4 grams of fiber.
- **Flaxseed**—These seeds have an impressive fiber content, with 2 tablespoons containing roughly 4 grams of fiber.

Whole psyllium husk is also a good fiber source. However, since some psyllium crops are sprayed with agricultural chemicals, it's best to purchase this fiber source in organic form to avoid health risks.

Pump Up the Probiotics

Probiotics are live, beneficial bacteria that populate your gut microbiome and help keep your gut healthy. You can consume probiotics through your food (which, as you know from other sections of this book, is my first choice), as well as through probiotic supplements.

Fermented foods are incredibly rich sources of probiotics. Although these foods were a mainstay of ancient cultures, as fermenting preserved them for later consumption, they've only relatively recently been embraced as a way to optimize gut health, but I'm certainly glad that they have. Each mouthful of fermented food can provide *trillions* of beneficial bacteria—*far* more than you can get from a probiotic supplement, which will typically provide you with colony-forming units in the billions. Fermented foods also give you a wider variety of beneficial bacteria than supplements do.

What specific foods am I talking about?

- **Fermented vegetables,** like cucumbers (pickles) and cabbage (sauerkraut and kimchi)
- **Kefir,** a fermented milk drink, much like yogurt
- **Miso**
- **Tempeh**
- **Natto,** a traditional Japanese fermented food made from soybeans
- **Raw yogurt from the milk of grass-fed animals** (most commercial varieties contain too much added sugar to be healthful choices; avoiding sugar in general is beneficial for your gut microbiome)

Note that many fermented foods on grocery store shelves, especially pickles and sauerkraut, don't contain live cultures. You want these items to be refrigerated, and make sure to read labels carefully to ensure you're getting alive, active probiotics. You can also ferment many foods at home, and the process is easier than you might think.

If you don't like fermented foods and don't eat a lot of them, you'll need to supplement with a probiotic on a regular basis, especially if you eat a lot of processed foods, as a poor diet can wipe out the beneficial bacteria in your gut, giving harmful pathogens free rein to proliferate.

But don't just grab the first supplement you see: Buy from a company with a good track record of making high-quality products that are manufactured following current Good Manufacturing Practices; look for a potency of 50 billion colony-forming units or higher; and select a supplement with multiple strains of probiotics. These supplements work best when taken on an empty stomach two hours before your first meal, or after the last meal of your day.

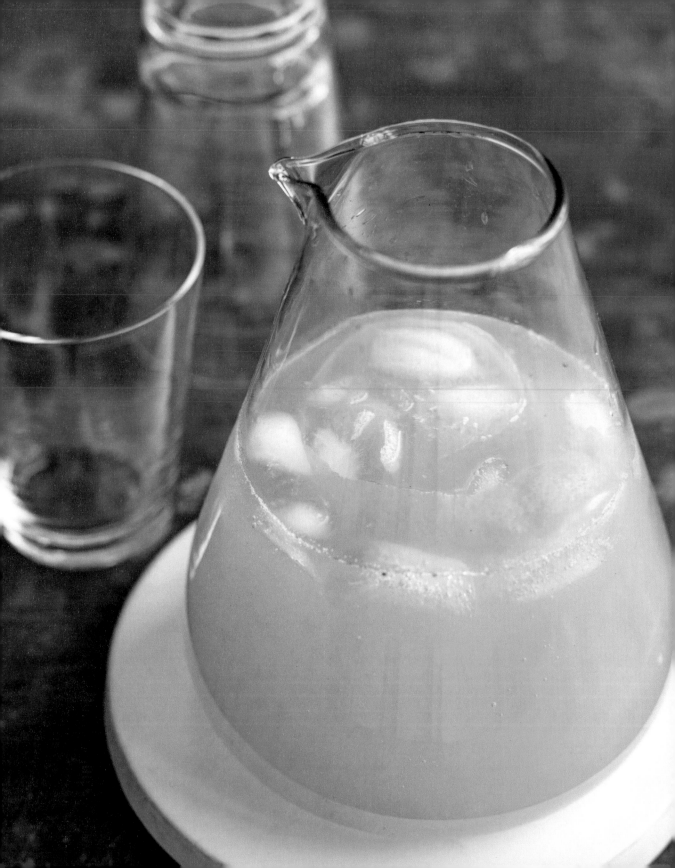

PROPER HYDRATION TIPS

Providing your body with proper hydration, especially in the form of pure water, is one of the simplest steps you can take to improve your overall health and boost your immunity. All your bodily systems rely on water to function optimally, which makes sense, as you're made up almost entirely of it: Your body contains about 42 liters of water, which accounts for up to 70 percent of your weight.

Your blood is a whopping 85 percent water, while your muscles and brain are close behind, at 80 percent and 75 percent, respectively. Water even makes up 25 percent of your bones. Your body needs water for blood circulation, metabolism, regulation of body temperature, waste removal, cognitive function, and a lot more.

When it comes to immunity specifically, water and other fluids:

- Aid in digestion, helping your body break down food and absorb its nutrients—the very nutrients that are crucial for a healthy immune system.

- Keep your mucous membranes moist, especially those in your mouth, nose, and eyes, which are your body's first-line defense against viruses and bacteria.

- Help lymph to move easily through your body; among other functions, your lymphatic system, as part of your immune system, produces immune cells including white blood cells, which protect your body from potentially harmful invaders.

- Flush any toxic invaders that do make their way into your body out, preventing buildup that could adversely affect your immune system.

A Look at the Research

Given all this, it should come as no surprise that countless studies link dehydration to disease and tie proper hydration to improved health outcomes. For example, high fluid intake is associated with a lower risk of certain types of cancer, including bladder, colorectal, and breast cancers. In one study, participants who drank the most fluid had a 49 percent lower incidence of bladder cancer than did those who drank the least.[1]

Scientists speculate that fluids may help combat cancer at least in part due to their ability to help maintain cell health and help the body eliminate cellular carcinogens. Other research suggests that as many as three million fewer Americans would suffer from degenerative diseases—including dementia, heart failure, and chronic lung disease—with improved hydration.[2]

How Much Water Should You Drink?

Despite the importance of adequate hydration, many children and adults don't drink enough water throughout the day, and it's estimated that as much as 30 percent of the elderly population may be dehydrated. It doesn't help that advice on how much water to consume is conflicting; also unhelpful is the lack of scientific evidence to back up the widespread advice to drink eight 8-ounce glasses of water a day. What's more, how much water a person needs is highly individual, based on one's age, body mass, pregnancy and breastfeeding status, diet, daily activities, and more.

So how can you determine the amount that's right for you? The good news is that your body will tell you. Once it has lost between 1 and 2 percent of its total water volume, your thirst mechanism will alert you that it's time to drink up. And using thirst as a guide is an easy and effective way to ensure your individual needs are met, day by day. Of course, if it's hot or exceptionally dry outside, or if you're engaged in exercise or other vigorous activity, you will require more water. But generally speaking, if you drink as soon as you feel thirsty, you should be able to remain well hydrated.

The color of your urine can also help you determine if you need to drink more water: If it is a deep, dark yellow, then you are likely not drinking enough. It should be a very light-colored, pale yellow. (Note that riboflavin, or vitamin B2, which is found in most multivitamins, turns urine a bright yellow.) If your urine is scant or if you haven't urinated in many hours, that too is an indication that you're not drinking enough. The results of several studies indicate that a healthy person urinates on average about seven or eight times a day. If you sleep eight hours a night, that means you're urinating approximately every two hours that you are awake.

Make Sure It's Filtered Water

Pure, clean water is the ideal beverage of choice for hydration. If you're on a community water system, don't just turn on the tap and fill a glass or water bottle, as it may very well contain fluoride, as well as heavy metals and disinfection by-products (DBPs) that can have ill effects on your health. Installing a water filter in your home, preferably both at the tap and at the point of entrance, can help eliminate these harmful contaminants.

As for the type of filtration system to get, there are a variety of options. A few of the most common include:

- **Reverse osmosis:** In addition to removing organic and inorganic contaminants (such as chlorine) from your water, reverse osmosis will remove about 80 percent of fluoride and most DBPs.

- **Ion exchange:** Such systems are designed to remove dissolved salts in your water, such as calcium. They also soften the water and help prevent the creation of scale buildup. The ion exchange system was originally used in boilers and other industrial applications before becoming popular in home water-purifying units, which usually combine the system with carbon filtering for greater effectiveness.

- **Granular carbon and carbon block filters:** These are the most common types of countertop and under-counter water filters. Granular activated carbon is recognized by the Environmental Protection Agency as the best available technology for the removal of organic chemicals like herbicides, pesticides, and industrial compounds. One of its downfalls is that the loose carbon material inside can channel, meaning that water can create pathways through it, thereby escaping filtering. Carbon block filters offer the same superior filtering ability but are compressed, with the carbon in a solid form. This eliminates channeling and gives makers the ability to precisely combine multiple media in a sub-micron filter cartridge.

Ideally, you should look for a filtration system that uses a combination of methods, as this will ensure the removal of the widest variety of contaminants. One good option is a family of filters that I believe are the best on the market in terms of effectiveness, value, and ease of use. They are all manufactured in the United States under exclusive contract with a company specializing in advanced water treatment products and include both countertop and under-counter models. (You can see them for yourself at mercolamarket.com by searching for Pure & Clear water filters.)

Tea Time

Tea is another great beverage choice, as it is not only water based and hydrating, but also abundant in antioxidant polyphenols, which promote immunity. In fact, tea appears to "prime" the immune system. In one investigation, the immune cells of tea drinkers responded five times faster to germs than did the immune cells of coffee drinkers; the researchers concluded that five cups of tea a day sharpened the body's disease-fighting capabilities.[3]

Tea in general appears to be associated with lower risk of cardiovascular disease and all-cause death. Green tea is perhaps the most researched tea, and studies indicate a wealth of health benefits, from decreased cancer risk to a reduced risk of depression, obesity, stroke, and bone thinning. Matcha is a healthy and tasty green tea choice. Black tea is also well studied—it contains antioxidant compounds that reduce damage inflicted by free radicals, and regular consumption has been shown to reduce risk of heart disease, lower blood sugar, and reduce levels of LDL (or "bad") cholesterol.[4]

In addition to these popular options, consider oolong, Darjeeling, and herbal selections like hibiscus, which is high in antioxidants as well as minerals and vitamin C. But beware of nonorganic teas that are grown in polluted environments. They can contain heavy metals or fluoride, which could lead to health issues. Instant tea may also contain excessive fluoride.

Other Options and What to Avoid

If you want to drink something more flavorful than water and aren't a big fan of tea, you can opt for raw, organic green juice made from fresh vegetables. I recommend refraining from juice with too many fruits, as it will have high amounts of sugar and calories. Go for a green juice recipe that combines one or two fruits with a larger amount of greens; just be careful not to overload on oxalates (see my note on page 40 about greens). That way, you can minimize your sugar intake and still get all the nutrients from the fruits and vegetables in their purest forms.

Know that in addition to fresh fruits and vegetables, certain foods like homemade broth provide valuable fluids too. As for sports drinks, the truth is they weren't created for the average person looking to address hydration needs—they were created for athletes and other highly active people who need extra energy and replenishment of electrolytes they may have lost through sweating. And indeed, they can be detrimental to your health, as they're often loaded with sugar. Other sweetened beverages, such as sodas and even commercial fruit juices, should also be avoided—they don't offer enough value to make them useful for hydrating purposes—as should energy drinks, which not only are high in sugar but can have dangerous levels of caffeine.

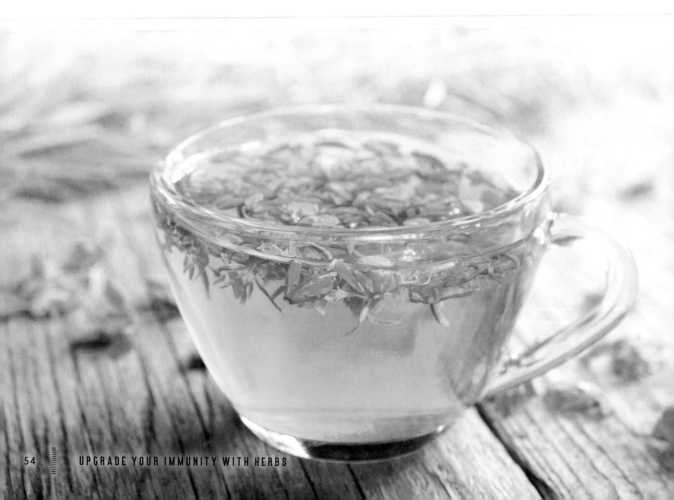

SLEEP STRATEGIES

Sleep is absolutely vital to your health—so critical, in fact, that no amount of prudent eating and exercise can counteract the ill effects of poor slumber. Depriving yourself of sleep dampens your immune system as much as physical stress or illness, which may explain why a lack of sleep is tied to an increased risk of so many chronic diseases, from Alzheimer's to cardiovascular disease to cancer. Fortunately, there are countless tips and tricks to help ensure you get a good night's rest.

Sick and Tired?

The evidence shows that sleep helps regulate the proliferation and activity of important immune cells, such as natural killer (NK) cells and T cells, and that it counteracts low-grade, systemic inflammation. In other words, it maintains immune homeostasis. You can think of it this way: Each night of sleep restores and readies your immune system for the next day.

Recent research has added to our understanding of sleep's impact on T cells in particular, which fight intracellular pathogens, including cells infected with viruses such as influenza, and cancer cells. When immune cells recognize a pathogenic cell, they activate a sticky protein called integrin, by which they attach themselves to the infected cell and ultimately destroy it.

In analyzing T cells from study participants when they slept through the night and when they stayed awake all night, researchers found that when participants slept, their T cells showed more integrin activation than when they were awake. And they figured out why: Certain stress hormones and pro-inflammatory molecules reduce the stickiness of integrin, and levels of these substances are lowest when the body is asleep. High levels from lack of sleep decrease the efficacy of T cells' immune response, while sleep helps enhance their efficiency in killing pathogens.[1]

This new understanding sheds light on findings from past studies on sleep and immunity. For example, one notable investigation studied 11 pairs of identical twins with different sleep habits (with one sleeping at least an hour less than the other, on average). Researchers gathered blood samples and found that the twin with the shorter nightly sleep duration had a depressed immune system relative to that of his or her sibling.[2]

In another, shorter sleep duration was associated with increased susceptibility to the common cold. Researchers collected data on the sleep patterns of more than 164 healthy men and women for one week, using wrist sensors and sleep diaries. Then they exposed these participants to rhinovirus (which causes the common cold) and monitored them over five days. They discovered that those who averaged five or six hours of sleep a night were four times more likely to catch a cold than were those who slept seven hours or more.[3]

In another, very similar study, researchers concluded that those who slept less than seven hours a night were three times more likely to develop a cold than those who slept eight hours or more. They also noted that those with reduced sleep efficiency (percentage of time actually asleep in bed) were more than five times as likely to come down with a cold as those with higher efficiency.[4] Other studies have shown similar results for pneumonia.

How Much Do You Need? Plus 11 Sleep Hacks

So, how many hours do you need a night? And what can you do to sleep longer and better? As a general rule, most adults need somewhere between seven and nine—or right around eight—hours of sleep a night to maintain good health. Here's how to get it.

Go to the dark side. Sleep in complete darkness, or as close to it as possible. Even the tiniest bit of light in the room, such as that from a clock radio screen, can interfere with your sleep. Get rid of night-lights, cover any screens, and use blackout shades or drapes; or consider a well-fitting sleep mask.

Monitor the temperature. Studies suggest the optimal room temperature for sleep is between 60 and 68 degrees—any higher or lower can have a negative impact. If your feet are cold, wear socks to bed or place a hot-water bottle near them. If you're hot, consider sleeping naked.

Eliminate EMFs. Electromagnetic fields from power sources in your bedroom can affect your body's production of melatonin and serotonin, which are involved in the sleep/wake cycle. One easy step to help reduce EMF exposure during sleep? Turn off your Wi-Fi at night. Also, move alarm clocks and other electronic devices away from your head, or preferably out of the room (this includes your cell phone). Avoid electric blankets. If you're able, shut down the electricity to your bedroom altogether by pulling your circuit breaker before bed.

Stick to a schedule. Go to bed and wake up at the same times each day, even on weekends. This will help your body get into a sleep rhythm and make it easier to fall asleep and wake up in the morning. Try to get to bed as early as possible, ideally between 9 and 10 P.M.

Make time to relax and unwind. Put your work away at least one hour before bed—preferably two hours or more—to give your mind a chance to unwind. Turn off the TV (see "Curb screen time," below) and establish a relaxing bedtime routine to release the tensions of the day. This can include meditation, reading, journaling, deep-breathing exercises, listening to relaxation CDs, or diffusing essential oils, as examples. Consider kicking off your nightly wind-down with a hot bath 90 to 120 minutes before bedtime. It's relaxing, and it increases your core body temperature; when you get out, your temperature drops and your body gets the message that it's about time to drift off. A hot shower can also be helpful.

Watch what you drink and eat. Avoid drinking anything within two hours of going to bed to reduce the likelihood of needing to get up and go to the bathroom, or at least minimize the frequency. (Be sure to go to the bathroom right before bed, too.) Likewise, avoid eating at least three hours before bedtime, particularly grains and sugars, which raise your blood sugar, delay sleep, and increase your risk of acid reflux. Of course, steer clear of any foods you're sensitive to. Also avoid caffeine later in the day (or altogether if it really affects you), as well as alcohol; although alcohol makes you drowsy, the effect is short lived, and it prevents you from entering the deep, restorative stages of sleep.

Curb screen time. Not only do electronic screens (TVs, phones, etc.) emit EMFs, they're major sleep thieves in general. The more time you spend on them during the day and especially at night, the longer it takes to fall asleep and the less sleep you end up getting. If you absolutely must use an electronic screen device late into the evening, wear blue-light-blocking glasses or install blue-blocking software; I have used Iris for many years.

Get moving. Exercising for at least 30 minutes per day can improve your sleep. However, don't exercise too close to bedtime (within three hours) or it may keep you awake. Studies show exercising in the morning is best if you can manage it. Exercising also helps you maintain a healthy weight; being overweight can increase your risk of sleep apnea, which can seriously impair your sleep.

Soak up the sun. Often, lack of sun exposure during the day (especially in the early morning) is to blame for persistent sleep problems.

Bright sunlight first thing in the morning and/or around solar noon helps set your internal clock, allowing you to fall asleep "on schedule."

Use your bed for . . . sleep and intimacy only. You want to create a clear association between your bed and sleep, not working or other activities.

Try EFT. My current favorite fix for insomnia is Emotional Freedom Techniques (EFT). Most people can learn the basics of this gentle tapping practice in a few minutes. EFT can help balance your body's bioenergy system and resolve some of the emotional stresses that contribute to insomnia at a very deep level.

Consider gentle sleep aids. Natural sleep remedies can help while you implement the lifestyle changes suggested above. Natural aids include these:

- *Melatonin.* Start with as little as 0.25 milligram and work your way up in quarter-milligram increments from there until you get the desired effect.

- *Valerian root.* Valerian can help you fall asleep faster and improve sleep quality. Start with a minimal dose and use the lowest dose needed to achieve the desired effect, as higher dosages can be energizing in some people. Typical dosages range between 400 and 900 mg, taken anywhere from 30 minutes to two hours before bed

- *Chamomile.* This herb is typically used in the form of infusions, teas, liquid extracts, or essential oils made from the plant's fresh or dried flower heads. It has sedative effects that may help with sleep, which is why chamomile tea is often sipped before bed; try incorporating it into your nightly relaxing routine (see above).

- *5-hydroxytryptophan (5-HTP)*. The chemical 5-HTP promotes production of serotonin, thereby giving mood a boost and enhancing sleep.

Help for Jet Lag

Sleep is easily affected by travel, especially when you're crossing time zones. As a general rule, your body will adjust to time zone changes at a rate of one day for each hour of time change. This means that if you need to be at your physical or psychological best on a particular day, you should travel as many days ahead of time as you'll need to adjust.

If you cannot squeeze in the extra time, you could act "as if" and pretend you're in your destination time zone while still at home. Simply wake up and go to bed according to the destination time rather than your local time, and be sure to shift your mealtimes accordingly. As an example, if you were planning to travel from New York to Paris, you would start going to bed (and shifting your mealtimes) an hour earlier each day, at least three days ahead of your flight (and as many as six days in advance, since there is a six-hour time difference between New York and Paris time), and avoid bright light for two to three hours before going to bed.

Here are a few other helpful pointers to consider:

- In the morning, be sure to expose yourself to bright, full-spectrum light.

If the sun is not yet up, use a clear incandescent lightbulb along with a cool-blue spectrum LED to shut down melatonin production.

- If traveling at night, wear blue-blocking glasses on the plane, and continue wearing them until you go to sleep, as excess blue light will impair your melatonin production and make it difficult to fall asleep.

- Once you're at your destination, get up as close to sunrise as possible and go outside. This will help to reset your melatonin production. If weather and circumstances allow, it's best to do this with your bare feet on the ground.

- At your destination, take a fast-acting sublingual dose of melatonin along with a slow-release oral melatonin around 10 P.M. (or just before bedtime if you go to bed earlier). Keep in mind that only a very small amount is required—typically 0.25 to 0.5 mg to start with; you can raise it from there. Taking higher doses, such as 3 mg, can sometimes make you more wakeful instead of sleepier, so adjust your dose carefully.

Most of this book so far has focused on what to add to your diet and healthy living routine to help improve your immunity—the beverages, herbs, spices, foods, and supplements that will shore up your system's defenses. However, what you exclude from your day-to-day life is equally important. Here is a list of things to avoid in order to keep your immune system in fighting shape.

Processed and Ultra-Processed Foods

If you could make only one change in your life to lower your risk of chronic disease, lose weight, and feel happier and more energized, you'd be well served to choose to reduce your intake of processed foods. You know that fast foods and refined junk foods aren't good for your body, as they're packed with sugar, synthetic and rancid fats, preservatives, genetically modified ingredients, additives, and other harmful elements.

This is especially the case for ultra-processed products, meaning foods that do not in any way resemble a food in its original form. This includes breakfast cereals, most commercial desserts, pizza, soda, packaged baked goods, microwavable frozen meals, instant soups and sauces, and chips and other salty, sweet, and savory snacks. Research has clearly shown that a high intake of these foods can lead to obesity (more below) as well as heart and kidney damage. Now we've come to understand that processed products damage the immune system, which may in part explain why these foods are also linked with an increased risk of cancer.

One way these foods harm your immunity is by weakening your gut microbiome and shifting the balance of bacteria there. (As discussed on pages 47–49, around 80 percent of your immune system resides in your gut.) Researchers point out that these immune impacts can be long lasting, as poor dietary choices get "encoded" into your gut and your genes and thus can get passed on to your offspring.[1]

A 2018 study echoes this observation. German researchers discovered not only that the immune system's inflammatory response to a fast-food diet is on par with the response it would give to a bacterial infection, but that this strong reaction persists. Even after the mice in the study were switched from processed foods to a healthy diet, their bodies' defenses remained hyperactive: Though acute inflammation disappeared, genes that had been switched on when the animals ate fast food were still active after a month, creating epigenetic changes that could in turn accelerate the development of diabetes and cardiovascular diseases.[2]

Any food that isn't directly from the vine, bush, tree, or earth is considered processed.

Not only do I encourage you to shun processed products in favor of fresh, whole foods, but I also encourage you to grow your own foods if you're in a position to do so. (Even if you don't have any outdoor space, you can grow herbs and sprouts on a sunny windowsill.) Homegrown food is usually more diverse, flavorful, and nutritious than processed foods bought from the store, retaining more of its vitamins, minerals, and antioxidants. Gardening also gets you exercising and reduces your stress levels, both of which I talk about in the pages ahead.

Alcohol

Various studies have linked excess alcohol consumption with an increased risk of chronic diseases such as pancreatitis and cancer—and, not surprisingly then, also with poor immune function. In fact, some research suggests that even moderate amounts of alcohol can negatively impact the immune response. Alcohol significantly increases inflammatory markers and compromises the structure and integrity of the gastrointestinal tract, altering the microbes in the gut that aid not only in normal gut function but also in immunity.

The science indicates that alcohol both disrupts the communication between gut microbes and the intestinal immune system and damages gut immune cells. Importantly, it also allows microbes to leak out of the gut. When they do, they end up in places like the liver and activate the innate immune system there, triggering inflammation that plays a role in alcoholic liver disease, which can lead to cirrhosis and liver cancer. In addition to promoting a proinflammatory response, alcohol also impairs an anti-inflammatory response from cytokines.

In general, researchers have found that alcohol interferes with the normal functioning of all aspects of the immune response and can negatively impact the numbers and function of all immune cell populations. Thus, chronic alcoholics have increased susceptibility to viral and bacterial infections.[3] Moderate alcohol intake is generally defined as no more than one drink a day for women and no more than two drinks a day for men. However, I recommend eliminating all alcohol if you're able, as it doesn't add much to an otherwise healthy diet and lifestyle and may indeed do harm.

Obesity

Of course, you want to maintain an appropriate weight for countless health reasons, not the least of which is an optimally functioning immune system. It turns out that there's a feedback loop in play when it comes to obesity and altered immunity: Obesity impairs the immune system, and an impaired immune system contributes to the development of obesity. Even obese individuals who eat a relatively healthy diet and exercise still appear to be at risk from impaired immune function.

While all the ways in which obesity and immunity are interconnected are not entirely clear, we do know that the disease reduces the production of cytokines and changes the way important immune cells such as lymphocytes (natural killer cells, T cells, and B cells), macrophages, and dendritic cells function, typically reducing their effectiveness.

Studies have found that obese hospitalized patients are more likely to develop secondary infections and complications such as pneumonia in the clinical setting, and that they tend to have longer stays when admitted to the ICU. Likewise, obesity seems to be a predictor for worse outcomes from the flu and is associated with increased risk for a number of bacterial infections.[4]

Fasting and time-restricted eating (within a six- to eight-hour eating window) can powerfully help obese individuals boost their fat burning and improve their metabolic efficiency and body composition, including reducing their visceral fat and body weight. I recommend my KetoFast protocol in particular, an approach that combines a cyclical ketogenic diet with intermittent fasting and cyclical partial fasting. Learn much more at my website, mercola.com, and in my book *KetoFast*.

Inactivity

Regular exercise does wonders for your immune system. It appears to give your immunity a boost in several ways: by acutely increasing your body temperature, which helps kill off invading pathogens (similar to the fever your body produces when you're sick); diversifying your gut microbiota, which in turn aids immune system functioning; and increasing the numbers of your immune cells.

When it comes to the latter, the science suggests that when you exercise at moderate to vigorous intensity, the activity stimulates the circulation of anti-inflammatory cytokines and immune cells such as T cells and natural killer cells. What's more, with regular exercise (near daily), these acute changes seem to add up to enhance your metabolic health and strengthen your immune system's defenses over time.[5]

This is evident in studies regarding exercise and the common cold. In one notable investigation, those who engaged in aerobic exercise five or more days a week cut their risk of developing a cold by nearly 50 percent when compared with those who were largely sedentary. What's more, those who exercised and did develop an infection experienced less severe symptoms.[6]

It's important to note, though, that some evidence points to immune dysfunction from intense exercise training, such as that undergone by competitors and athletes. Habits take time to form and time to break. If you've never exercised before, it's important to start slowly and build for long-lasting results, and to find the type of exercise you enjoy, so that doing it reduces your stress level and increases the likelihood you'll establish a regular routine.

You may want to begin with daily walks and build from there. Once walking has become routine, consider incorporating body-weight exercises or resistance bands. You can also add strength training using body-weight exercises that do not require any equipment.

Unnecessary Medications

The list of over-the-counter and prescription drugs that weaken your immune system is quite long. While there may be drugs you absolutely need to take, I encourage you to avoid unnecessary medications, particularly antibiotics, which are overprescribed and so often given for viral infections that will never respond to these drugs. We know that antibiotics have short- and long-term effects on the composition and health of your gut microbiome, which plays a crucial role in your overall immune function and general health.

Be careful as well with nonprescription drugs like cold- and fever-fighting medications, which can also have a negative impact on your immune system—the exact opposite of what you want when you're trying to fight a virus. Focus on the immune-boosting strategies shared throughout these pages before popping a pill.

Stress

There's a statistic floating around out there that as much as 90 percent of all diseases and illnesses can be attributed to stress. While we don't actually have an exact number, stress certainly does play a huge role in your overall health and well-being and has a major influence on the function of your immune system, which is why you've probably noticed you're more likely to catch a cold when you're under a lot of stress.

This is true for both acutely stressful episodes, such as preparing a big project for work, and chronic stress, such as relationship troubles or grief. Both will deteriorate your immune system and leave it less able to fight off infection. Indeed, in one study, participants who reported being under stress were twice as likely as unstressed subjects to get sick when infected with the virus that causes the common cold.[7]

Researchers have shown that the stress hormone cortisol may play an intricate role in the way high levels of stress are so detrimental to your immune system. When you're stressed, your body releases cortisol and other hormones that prepare your body to fight or flee the stressful event. Your heart rate increases, your lungs take in more oxygen, your blood flow increases, and parts of your immune system become

temporarily suppressed, which reduces your inflammatory response to pathogens. When stress becomes chronic, however, your immune system becomes less sensitive to cortisol, actually heightening the inflammatory response.

There are numerous ways to combat stress. Here are some of my favorite stress-reduction methods:

- **Meditation.** There are many different approaches to meditation. Mindfulness meditation in particular is a simple tool that's scientifically proven to relieve stress. Once you learn how to do it, you can practice it anytime, anywhere. You can turn to a mindfulness training program, or you can give it a go yourself at home with no formal training. Simply sit quietly (perhaps with some soothing music playing), breathe rhythmically, and focus on your breath or a flower, an image, a candle, a mantra, or even on just being there, fully aware, in the moment. I enjoy using Muse, which is a personal meditation assistant that promotes relaxation and even provides real-time feedback on how well you're doing. Personally, I find my best meditation time is in the morning, right after I awaken, as I can get into the deepest states of relaxation then.

- **Massage.** There's no denying that a massage can be wonderfully relaxing. Consider an aromatherapy lymph drainage massage specifically. Scents from essential oils such as lavender can be great stress relievers, and lymphatic massage itself boosts your immunity. Your lymphatic system produces, stores, and carries white blood cells that your body uses to fight off infections and disease, and lymphatic vessels branch out into all the tissues in your body, similar to blood vessels. Lymphatic fluid, or lymph, carries white blood cells throughout your body and also carries bacteria and toxins to your lymph nodes, where your immune system destroys them.

- **Laughter.** Laughter is seriously good medicine. It actually lowers levels of stress hormones in the body, among numerous other health benefits. There are lots of ways to get more laughter into your day: Watch comedies and read funny books, spend time with friends who make you happy and make you laugh, and remind yourself to play and have fun.

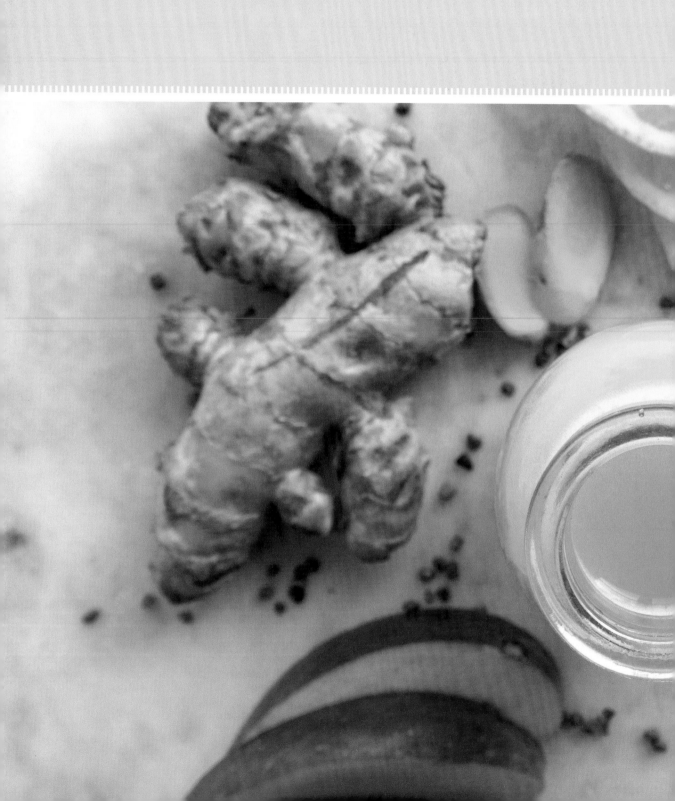

PART II

IMMUNE-BOOSTING RECIPES

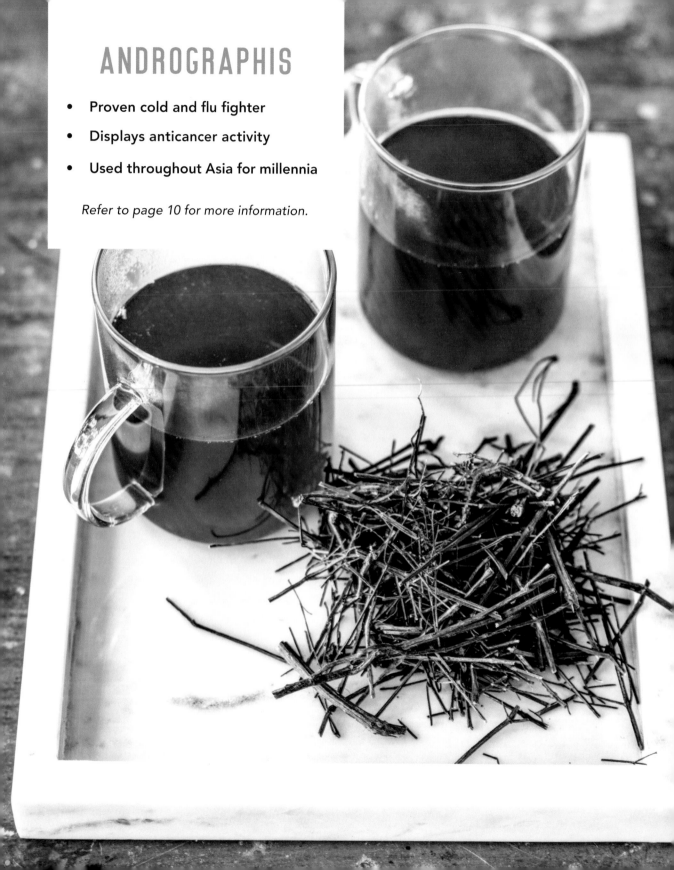

ANDROGRAPHIS

- Proven cold and flu fighter
- Displays anticancer activity
- Used throughout Asia for millennia

Refer to page 10 for more information.

IMMUNITY-BOOSTING ANDROGRAPHIS TEA

Drinking this at the first sign that you're coming down with something can help shorten the duration of a viral infection and reduce the severity of symptoms. But don't wait until you detect that telltale tickle in your throat—add this to your regular tea rotation during cold and flu season and it will help you ward off any invaders from taking root in the first place. Because andrographis is a bit bitter, the honey really helps this natural medicine go down.

1. Place all the ingredients in a bowl and mix to combine.

2. Transfer the mixture to an airtight container and store in the pantry for up to 1 month.

3. For each cup of tea, steep 1 teaspoon of andrographis tea in 1 cup of boiling water until cool enough to drink.

4. Strain into a mug, add a little manuka honey for some sweetness, and sip slowly.

NOTE: You can find andrographis stems, echinacea, ginger root, licorice root, and elderflower in health food stores, specialty tea shops, some supermarkets, and online.

Serves: 6

1 tablespoon andrographis stems

1 tablespoon dried echinacea leaves

2 teaspoons dried ginger root

2 teaspoons licorice root

2 teaspoons dried elderflower

Organic manuka honey, to taste

NUTRITION INFORMATION: Nutrition information for this recipe is not readily available

ASHWAGANDHA SLEEP TONIC

One of the biggest problems of stress is that it can prevent you from getting a good night's sleep, which is when your body renews itself and deals with the tensions of the previous day and prepares for the day ahead. This tonic has not only lavender and chamomile to take the edge off your stress, but also ashwagandha, an adaptogen, which provides your body with just what it needs to recuperate from the stress. And when you're rested, everything works better—your brain, your nervous system, your metabolism, and your immunity.

Serves: 2

1 vanilla pod, split, and seeds scraped and reserved

2 cinnamon sticks

5 cardamom pods, bruised

¼ teaspoon fennel seeds

1 star anise

2 whole cloves

1 teaspoon dried lavender

2 teaspoons dried chamomile

½ to 1 teaspoon ashwagandha root powder

¾ cup hemp milk, or milk of your choice such as coconut, macadamia, or almond milk

TO SERVE

1 to 2 teaspoons manuka honey, or to your liking (optional)

1 to 2 small pinches of ground cinnamon

1. Bring 1½ cups of water to a boil in a saucepan.

2. Reduce the heat to low. Add the vanilla pod and scraped vanilla seeds, the spices, and the dried lavender and chamomile, and gently simmer for 15 minutes to allow the flavors to develop. Stir in the ashwagandha powder and hemp milk and warm over low heat until the milk is heated through.

3. Pour the hot liquid through a fine strainer into a heat-proof jar or teapot, then transfer to two mugs.

4. Stir some manuka honey into the sleep tonic for some sweetness, if desired, and finish with a pinch of ground cinnamon.

NUTRITION INFORMATION: Calories 349.2 | 11.5g total fat (2.1g saturated fat, 0g trans fat) | 0mg cholesterol | 255mg sodium | 52.7g total carbohydrate (13.6g dietary fiber, 6.7g total sugars, 0g added sugars) | 12.7g protein | 1.3mcg vitamin D | 430.1mg calcium | 21mg iron | 266.6mg potassium

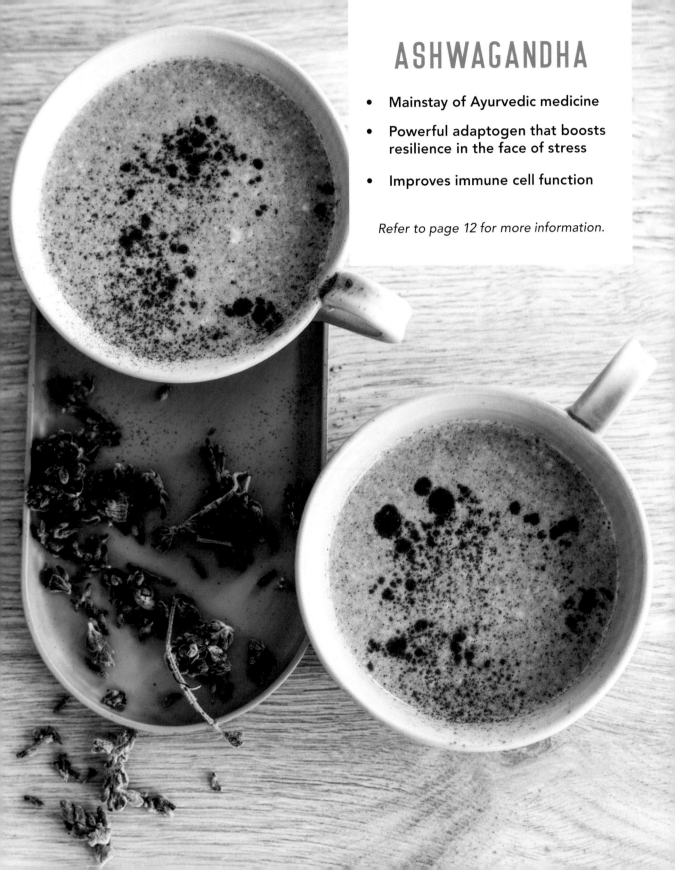

ASHWAGANDHA

- Mainstay of Ayurvedic medicine
- Powerful adaptogen that boosts resilience in the face of stress
- Improves immune cell function

Refer to page 12 for more information.

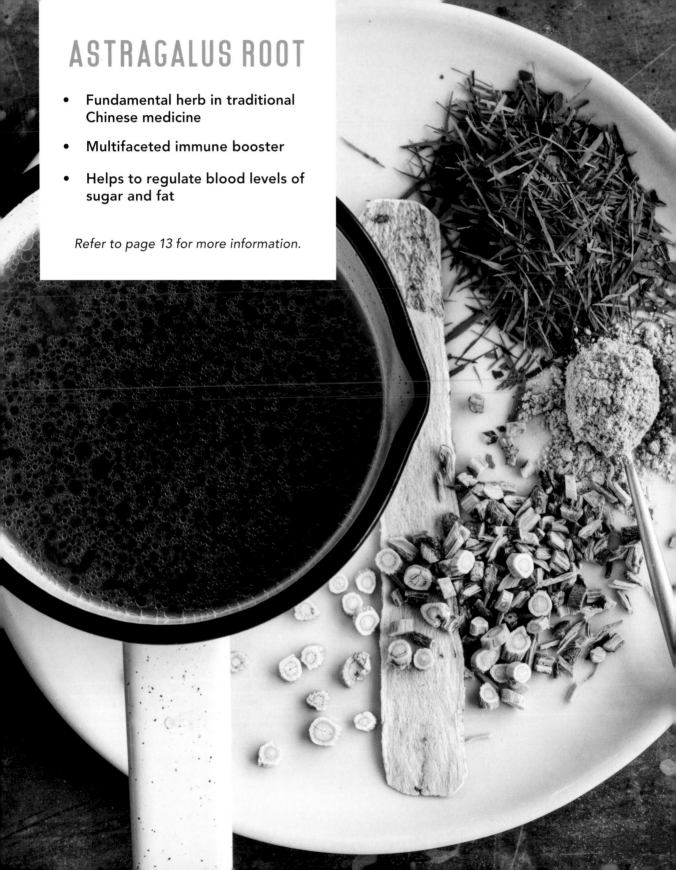

ASTRAGALUS ROOT

- Fundamental herb in traditional Chinese medicine

- Multifaceted immune booster

- Helps to regulate blood levels of sugar and fat

Refer to page 13 for more information.

ASTRAGALUS ROOT BROTH
WITH LICORICE

Drinking this nourishing broth is like taking your immune system to the gym: Thanks to the astragalus, licorice root, pau d'arco (an anti-inflammatory and antimicrobial), and slippery elm (used to treat a range of ailments, from coughs to diarrhea), it's a great immune strengthener. Combining these immunity powerhouses with bone broth helps to improve gut health, which also benefits immunity, as 80 percent of your immune system is located in the gut. You can buy beef bone broth at most health food markets, or use my recipe for it in the *KetoFast Cookbook*.

1. Place the beef bone broth in a medium saucepan, stir in the astragalus, licorice root, and pau d'arco bark, cover, and bring to a boil.

2. Remove the mixture from the heat, stir in the slippery elm, and allow it to steep for 1 hour.

3. Strain the liquid into a glass jar and store it in the fridge. Or if you would like to drink it right away, reheat the broth in a saucepan, add a pinch of sea salt to taste, pour into mugs, and enjoy!

Serves: 4

4 cups beef bone broth

¼ cup astragalus root slices

¼ cup licorice root

2 tablespoons pau d'arco bark

1 teaspoon slippery elm powder

Sea salt

NUTRITION INFORMATION: Calories 90.7 | 0.1g total fat (0.1g saturated fat, 0g trans fat) | 0mg cholesterol | 242.4mg sodium | 23.3g total carbohydrate (9.1g dietary fiber, 2.3g total sugars, 0.1g added sugars) | 2.3g protein | 0mcg vitamin D | 193.7mg calcium | 0.2mg iron | 110.7mg potassium

CHYAWANPRASH JAM

Hugely popular in India and hailed in Ayurvedic medicine, this herb-infused gooseberry jam is said to restore your life force and delay aging. I like stirring 1 or 2 teaspoons into a small cup of warmed hemp milk, or you can use it as you would any other jam. It's a great morning tonic you can take year round, or primarily in the colder months.

Makes: 4 servings

3 cups gooseberries, tops and stems removed

1 bay leaf

1 tablespoon dried ginger

8 cardamom pods

1½ tablespoons black peppercorns

1 cinnamon stick

1 tablespoon cumin seeds

1 tablespoon fennel seeds

10 whole cloves

20 threads saffron

1 teaspoon ground nutmeg

1 cup ghee or coconut oil

1½ cups coconut sugar

1 cup raw organic honey

1. Place the gooseberries in a medium saucepan filled with water and bring to a boil. Reduce to a simmer and cook for 15 minutes or until the gooseberries are very tender.

2. Strain out the liquid through a colander and allow the berries to cool slightly.

3. When cool enough to handle, remove and discard the seeds, then place the gooseberry flesh in a bowl and mash with a potato masher into a smooth paste. You can also use a food processor and blend until smooth. Set aside.

4. Place all the spices, excluding the ground nutmeg, in a spice grinder and grind into a fine powder. Mix in the nutmeg and set aside.

5. Heat the ghee in a large saucepan over medium heat. Stir in the coconut sugar and mix until the sugar has dissolved.

6. Reduce the heat to medium-low, then add the gooseberry paste. Mix to combine, then cook, stirring occasionally, for 8 to 10 minutes or until the mixture darkens and is reduced to a thick paste.

7. Add the spice mixture and cook, stirring frequently, for 2 minutes or until fragrant.

8. Remove from heat and allow to cool completely.

9. Once the mixture has cooled, mix in the raw organic honey to combine.

10. Transfer to glass jars with lids or airtight containers, and store in the fridge for up to 6 months.

NUTRITION INFORMATION: Calories 722 | 36.2g total fat (21.4g saturated fat, 1.4g trans fat) | 87.5mg cholesterol | 82.9mg sodium | 100.4g total carbohydrate (7.9g dietary fiber, 79.1g total sugars, 0.7g added sugars) | 3.9g protein | 0.1mcg vitamin D | 104.6mg calcium | 2.8mg iron | 417.7mg potassium

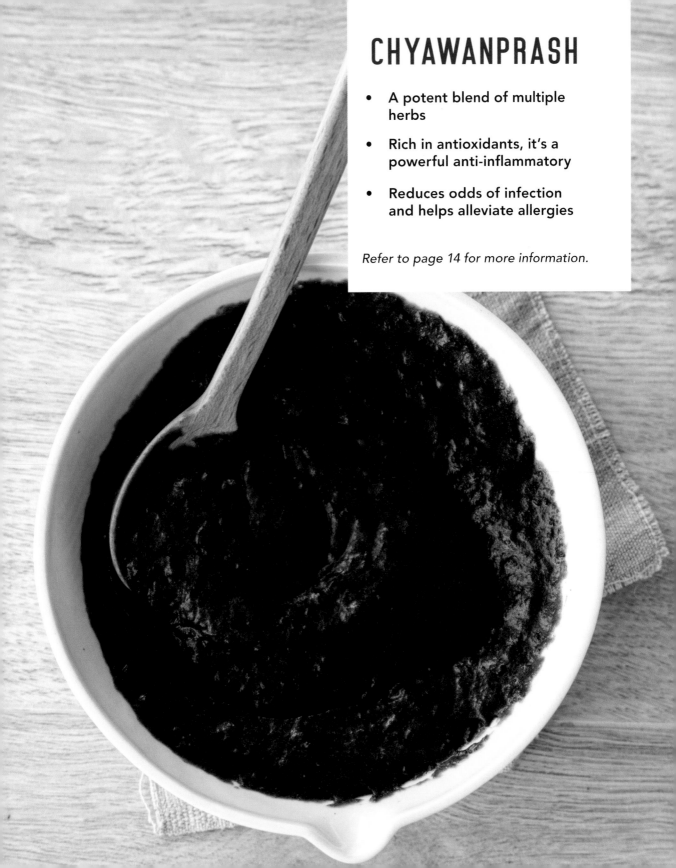

CHYAWANPRASH

- A potent blend of multiple herbs

- Rich in antioxidants, it's a powerful anti-inflammatory

- Reduces odds of infection and helps alleviate allergies

Refer to page 14 for more information.

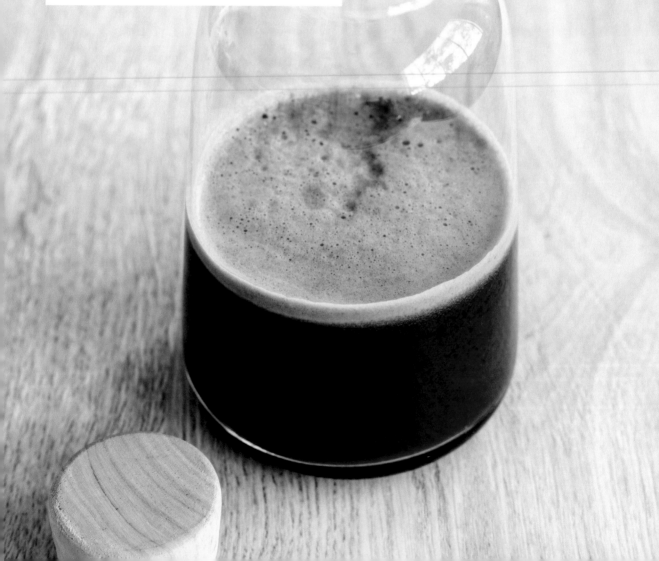

DANDELION

- Hailed worldwide for its medicinal properties

- Anti-inflammatory, antibacterial, antiviral, and anticancer

- Strong body of evidence to support its effectiveness in a wide range of conditions and diseases

Refer to page 17 for more information.

ALOE VERA AND DANDELION LEAF JUICE

This green juice will recharge your batteries! The aloe vera promotes hydration and elimination, the cilantro helps usher toxins out of your body, and the dandelion greens are an all-around tonic. Moringa and graviola—two immune-enhancing herbs—amp up the benefit of this juice, but it's still a powerhouse without them, so give it a try even if you don't have them on hand.

1. Juice the dandelion, parsley, cilantro, cucumber, lemon, and Swiss chard, then stir in the aloe and the moringa and graviola (if using).

2. Pour into two tall glasses and serve immediately.

Serves: 2

4 large handfuls dandelion leaves

1 handful parsley leaves

1 handful cilantro leaves

1 cucumber

½ lemon

4 Swiss chard leaves and stalks

⅓ cup aloe vera leaf juice

1 teaspoon moringa (optional)

1 teaspoon graviola (optional)

NUTRITION INFORMATION: Calories 106.2 | 1.4g total fat (0.3g saturated fat, 0g trans fat) | 0mg cholesterol | 509.3mg sodium | 55.9g total carbohydrate (9.5g dietary fiber, 4.2g total sugars, 0g added sugars) | 7.3g protein | 0mcg vitamin D | 307.1mg calcium | 5mg iron | 175mg potassium

ECHINACEA TEA

The natural health movement opened up a whole world of teas that can be brewed from different plants and their leaves, roots, flowers, buds, stalks, and pollen—and even, in some instances, the resin formed between rocks. There is certainly more to tea than the Lipton so many of us grew up with! I invite you to enjoy a cup of this echinacea brew anytime you feel your resilience needs a lift.

NOTE: Echinacea can be a problem for some people with autoimmune disease, so please consult your health care provider to learn more.

Serves: 10

2 tablespoons echinacea leaves

1 cinnamon stick, broken into small pieces

1 tablespoon dried rose hips

1 tablespoon dandelion tea leaves (see note on page 17)

1 teaspoon finely grated fresh turmeric or ½ teaspoon ground turmeric

1. Place all the ingredients in a bowl and mix to combine.

2. Transfer the mixture to an airtight container and store in the pantry for up to 1 month.

3. For each cup of tea, add 2 teaspoons of the tea blend to 1 cup of boiling water and steep until cool enough to drink.

4. Strain into a mug and sip slowly.

NOTE: You can find echinacea leaves and dried rose hips in health food stores, specialty tea shops, and some supermarkets, or online.

NUTRITION INFORMATION: Nutrition information for this recipe is not readily available

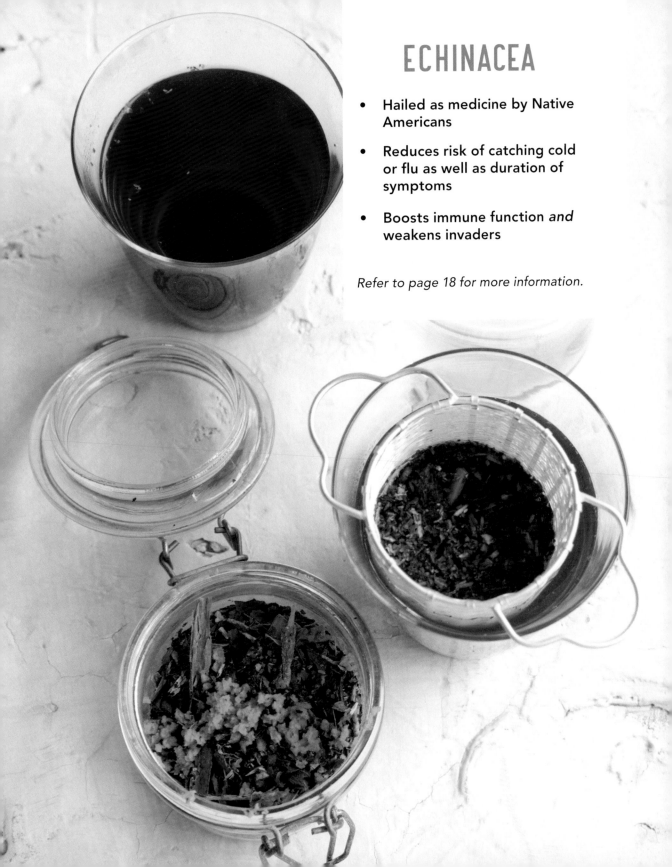

ECHINACEA

- Hailed as medicine by Native Americans

- Reduces risk of catching cold or flu as well as duration of symptoms

- Boosts immune function *and* weakens invaders

Refer to page 18 for more information.

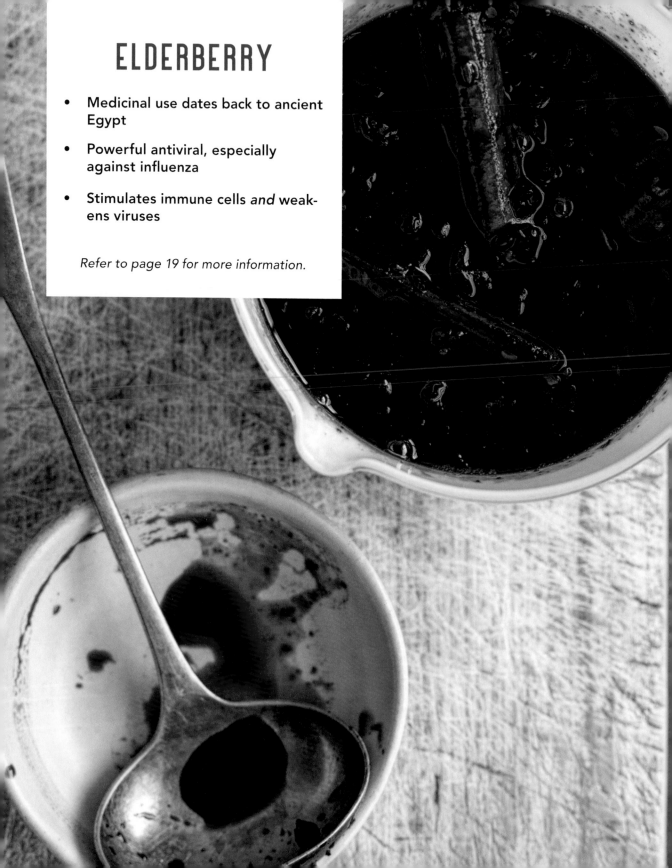

ELDERBERRY

- Medicinal use dates back to ancient Egypt

- Powerful antiviral, especially against influenza

- Stimulates immune cells *and* weakens viruses

Refer to page 19 for more information.

ELDERBERRY SYRUP

Here's an immune booster that your kids will happily swallow down. It will help everyone in your household stay virus free—even during those early years when it feels as if the kids are bringing some new bug home every week. Take 1 to 2 teaspoons a day during cold and flu season to keep your immunity strong; you can also take that dosage twice a day if you feel you're coming down with something to amp up its antiviral, antibiotic, and antimicrobial effects.

1. Place 4 cups of water in a medium saucepan. Add the elderberries, ginger, cinnamon sticks, and cloves and stir to combine.

2. Bring to a boil over medium heat, then turn down to medium-low and gently simmer for 1 hour, stirring occasionally, or until the liquid is reduced by almost half.

3. Remove from the heat and allow to cool slightly.

4. When cool enough to handle, remove and discard the cinnamon sticks.

5. Pass the berry mixture through a sieve into a bowl, pressing with the back of a spoon to release as much liquid as possible. Discard the leftover elderberry pulp and cloves.

6. Add the honey to the warm elderberry mixture and stir well to form a lovely syrup.

7. Pour the syrup into a mason jar or glass bottle with a fitted screw-top lid and store in the fridge for up to 3 months.

Makes: 2 cups

1 cup dried elderberries

3 tablespoons finely grated ginger

2 cinnamon sticks

3 whole cloves

1½ cups raw honey

NUTRITION INFORMATION: Calories 38.5 | 0.2g total fat (0g saturated fat, 0g trans fat) | 0mg cholesterol | 3.6mg sodium | 10.4g total carbohydrate (0.6g dietary fiber, 8.5g total sugars, 0g added sugars) | 0.1g protein | 0mcg vitamin D | 6.4mg calcium | 0.2mg iron | 25.3mg potassium

SAUTÉED LAMB
WITH RED ONION AND HERB SALAD

This flavorful dish will make your taste buds and your immune system happy (the garlic in particular is a potent antiviral). Sumac is a bright-red Middle Eastern spice that delivers a citrusy brightness *and* antiseptic powers to any dish. It's optional in this recipe, but it's worth seeking out and adding to your spice cabinet; I think you'll find yourself reaching for it again and again to season meats, vegetable dishes, and even sweet treats. Harissa is a North African spicy chili paste that's available in many gourmet or international markets; it adds a delicious kick.

Serves: 4

1⅓ pounds lamb fillets or lamb liver, cut into ¾-inch-thick strips

1 tablespoon harissa

3 garlic cloves, finely grated

⅓ cup melted coconut oil or good-quality animal fat

Freshly ground black pepper

⅓ cup very thinly sliced red onion

¼ cup pomegranate seeds

½ teaspoon sumac (optional)

1 large lemon slice, to serve

SAFFRON YOGURT

12 saffron threads

¾ cup coconut yogurt

Sea salt

DRESSING

2 teaspoons lemon juice

½ teaspoon Dijon mustard

2 tablespoons extra-virgin olive oil

HERB SALAD

2 handfuls mint leaves

2 handfuls cilantro leaves

1. Place the lamb, harissa, garlic, and 2 tablespoons of the coconut oil in a bowl and mix well. Cover and marinate in the fridge for 1 hour or, even better, overnight.

2. To make the saffron yogurt, place 1 tablespoon of warm water in a small bowl, add the saffron threads, and set aside to soak for 10 minutes. (Hydrating the saffron threads brings out their gorgeous floral flavor, color, and aroma.) Add the coconut yogurt and a pinch of salt and mix well.

3. Heat the remaining coconut oil in a large, heavy frying pan over medium-high heat. Season the marinated lamb with salt and pepper and fry in batches, tossing frequently, for 5 to 6 minutes or until pink in the middle (or cooked to your liking). Transfer the lamb to a bowl and let it rest for a few minutes, keeping it warm.

4. Combine the dressing ingredients in a bowl and whisk until emulsified. Season with salt and pepper.

5. To make the herb salad, combine the mint and coriander in a bowl, add the dressing, and gently toss.

6. Arrange the lamb on a serving platter, add the herb salad, and drizzle any dressing remaining in the bowl over the salad and lamb. Dollop some saffron yogurt onto the lamb, scatter the red onion and pomegranate seeds over it, and sprinkle on the sumac, if using. Serve with a lemon slice on the side.

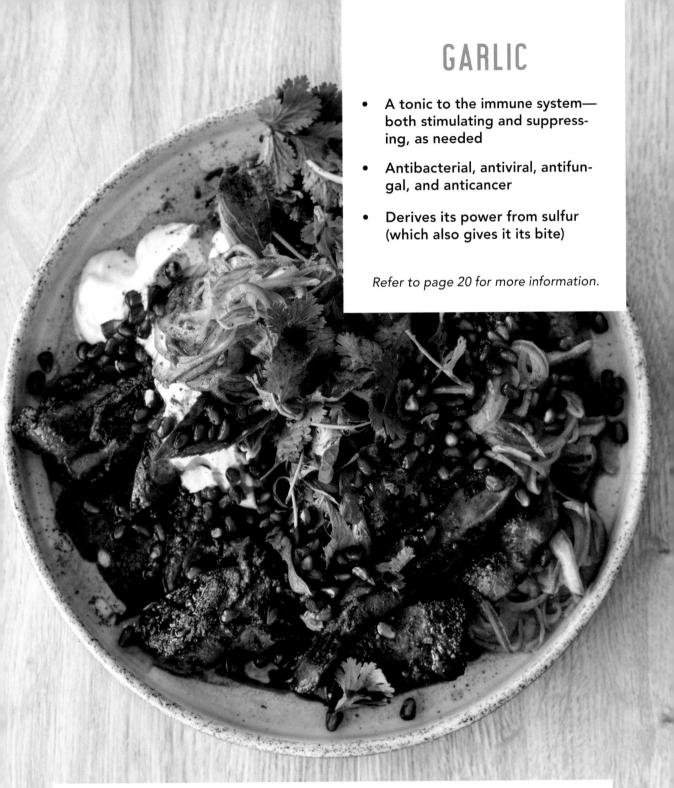

GARLIC

- A tonic to the immune system—both stimulating and suppressing, as needed

- Antibacterial, antiviral, antifungal, and anticancer

- Derives its power from sulfur (which also gives it its bite)

Refer to page 20 for more information.

NUTRITION INFORMATION: Calories 704.9 | 44.8g total fat (25.8g saturated fat, 0g trans fat) | 876.8mg cholesterol | 299.5mg sodium | 17.5g total carbohydrate (1.9g dietary fiber, 3.9g total sugars, 0g added sugars) | 55.8g protein | 0.9mcg vitamin D | 48.1mg calcium | 18.2mg iron | 650.2mg potassium

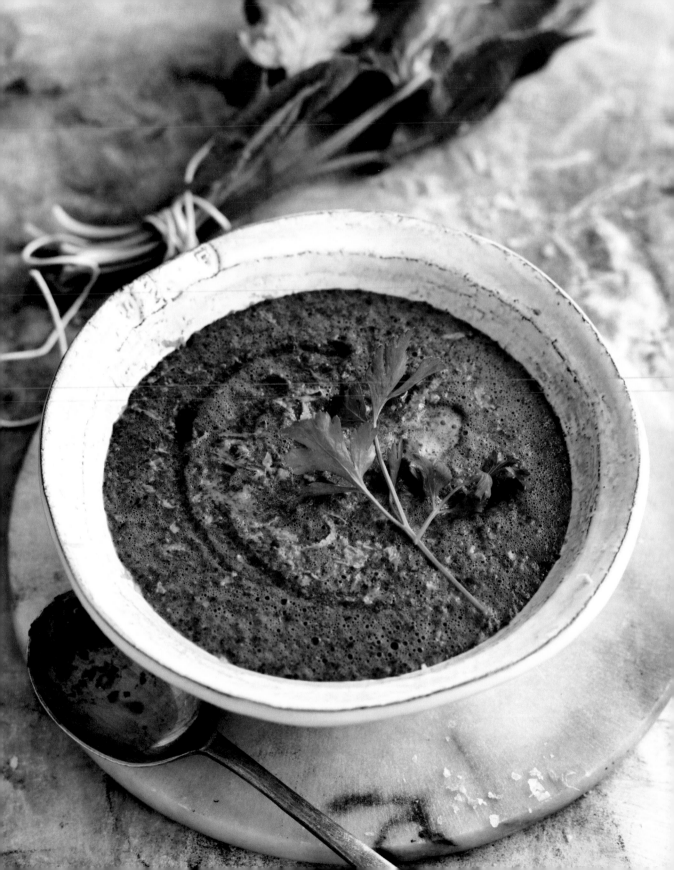

CHICKEN BROTH
WITH WATERCRESS AND LEMON

This is the perfect dish to include in your diet, especially if you are considering doing a fast. I sometimes heat up my broth, add a particular in-season vegetable, and cook it until tender, then blend it to create a wonderful variation on this soup. You might like to try mushrooms, broccoli, zucchini, cauliflower, okra, asparagus, onion, Jerusalem artichoke, parsnip, and sweet potato (just go easy on the starchy vegetables if you want to stay low carb).

1. Bring the broth to a boil in a large saucepan over medium-high heat. Reduce the heat to low, add the onion and garlic, and simmer for 15 minutes or until the onion is tender. Add the watercress and parsley and cook for 2 minutes.

2. Using a handheld blender, blend the soup until smooth. Season with salt and pepper to taste, then stir in the lemon juice.

3. Ladle the soup into serving bowls, sprinkle the lemon zest over the top, and drizzle with some olive oil. Garnish with an extra sprig of parsley.

Serves: 4

4 cups Chicken Bone Broth (page 146)

½ onion, chopped

4 garlic cloves, chopped

¾ cup roughly chopped watercress

1 large handful flat-leaf parsley leaves, plus extra sprigs for serving

Sea salt and freshly ground black pepper

1 tablespoon lemon juice

1 teaspoon finely grated lemon zest

Extra-virgin olive oil, to serve

NUTRITION INFORMATION: Calories 73.6 | 4.2g total fat (0.7g saturated fat, 0g trans fat) | 0.7mg cholesterol | 139.6mg sodium | 6.8g total carbohydrate (0.9g dietary fiber, 2.5g total sugars, 0g added sugars) | 2.8g protein | 0mcg vitamin D | 59.3mg calcium | 0.4mg iron | 250.3mg potassium

ROASTED TROUT
WITH JERK SPICE GLAZE

Spices can transform the humblest of ingredients into superstars. Jamaican jerk spice combines thyme, garlic, and some of the world's most intoxicating and addictive spices—allspice, cloves, cinnamon, and nutmeg—with the heat of chiles. Try adding this spice mix to your next meatloaf or Bolognese sauce, or rub it onto a chicken before roasting.

NOTE: Always try to source local, sustainable seafood.

Serves: 6

Melted coconut oil, for brushing

6 trout fillets (about 6 ounces each), skin left on, pin bones removed

Salt and pepper

Herb and Anchovy Dressing (see recipe on page 157)

JERK SPICE GLAZE

3 spring onions, finely chopped

2 garlic cloves, finely chopped

1 habanero or Scotch bonnet chile, seeded and finely chopped

3 tablespoons molasses

2 tablespoons coconut sugar

2 tablespoons tamari

1½ tablespoons coconut oil, melted

1½ tablespoons dark rum (optional)

½ tablespoon lemon juice

½ tablespoon dried thyme

½ teaspoon ground allspice

¼ teaspoon ground cinnamon

Pinch of freshly grated nutmeg

½ teaspoon sea salt

¼ teaspoon freshly ground black pepper

1. Position a rack in the center of the oven and preheat the oven to 400 °F. Line a baking tray with foil and brush with coconut oil.

2. To make the jerk spice glaze, place all of the glaze ingredients in a food processor bowl and pulse until blended. Pour the mixture into a small bowl and set aside.

3. Pat each trout fillet dry with paper towels, then season with salt and pepper to taste. Place the trout, skin side down, on the prepared tray.

4. Generously brush the top of the trout with the jerk spice glaze, then roast for 6 to 8 minutes or until the flesh is tender and opaque.

5. Place a piece of trout on each of 6 serving plates and top with 2 tablespoons of herb and anchovy dressing. Serve with your favorite salad.

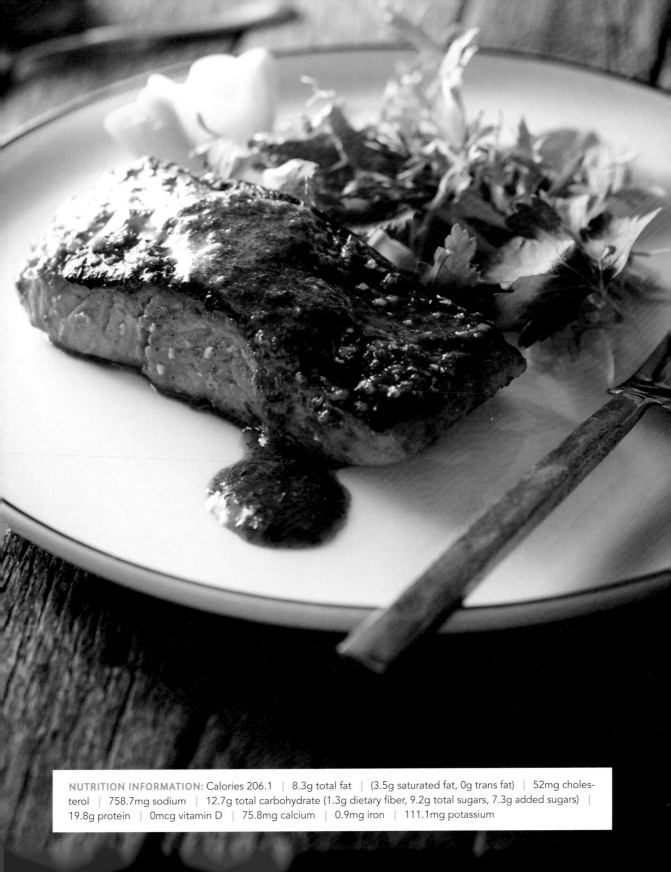

NUTRITION INFORMATION: Calories 206.1 | 8.3g total fat | (3.5g saturated fat, 0g trans fat) | 52mg cholesterol | 758.7mg sodium | 12.7g total carbohydrate (1.3g dietary fiber, 9.2g total sugars, 7.3g added sugars) | 19.8g protein | 0mcg vitamin D | 75.8mg calcium | 0.9mg iron | 111.1mg potassium

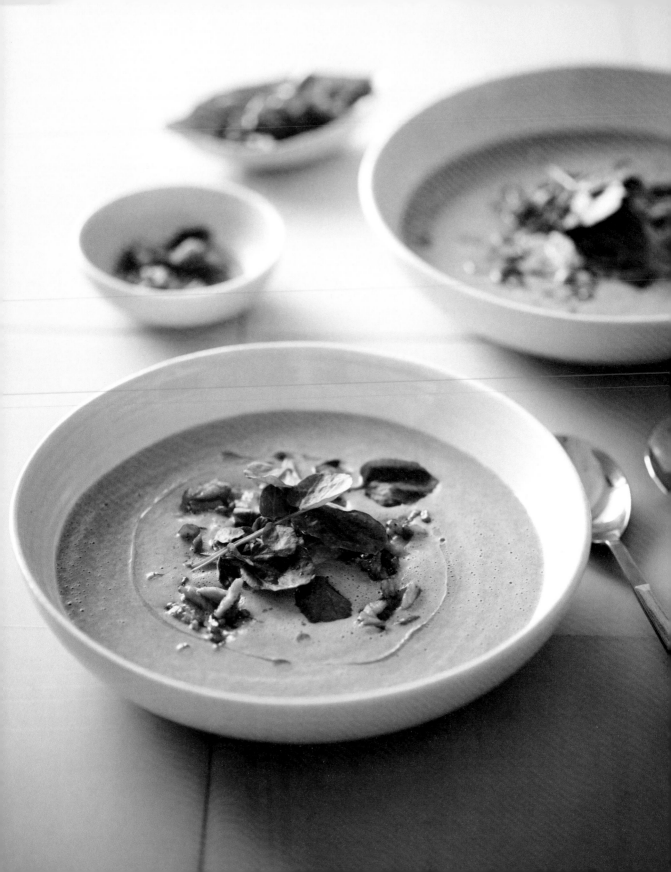

CHICKEN LIVER SOUP WITH CRISPY BACON AND WATERCRESS

We should be eating a lot more organ meats, especially liver, as it is a superfood. This nourishing chicken broth flavored with bacon, mushrooms, thyme, and liver is a luxurious and medicinal meal fit for a queen or king.

1. Melt the coconut oil in a saucepan over medium heat. Add the onion and cook, stirring occasionally, for 8 minutes or until softened and starting to caramelize. Stir in the garlic and cook for 1 minute or until fragrant.

2. Add the livers and cook for 3 minutes or until browned but still pink inside. Remove the livers from the pan and set aside. Add the mushrooms and thyme to the pan, pour in the broth, and bring to a boil. Reduce the heat to low and simmer for 10 minutes, stirring occasionally.

3. Meanwhile, preheat the oven to 400 °F. Place the bacon on a baking tray and cook in the oven for 4 to 5 minutes. Flip the bacon and cook for a further 4 to 5 minutes or until golden brown and crisp. When cool enough to handle, chop the bacon into small pieces.

4. Return the chicken livers to the pan and cook for 3 minutes.

5. Season with salt and pepper to taste. Blend the soup with a handheld blender until smooth. Add more broth if desired.

6. Ladle the soup into warm serving bowls, sprinkle with the bacon crisps, and top with the watercress. Finish with a drizzle of extra-virgin olive oil.

NOTE: If you use half the amount of broth in this recipe, this soup becomes a wonderful pâté. Simply place in ramekins and chill in the fridge until set. Serve with veggie sticks and seeded crackers.

Serves: 3 to 4

2 tablespoons coconut oil or good-quality animal fat

1 large onion, chopped

4 garlic cloves, chopped

1 pound organic chicken livers, sinew removed (or use duck, lamb, or beef liver)

8 ounces mushrooms (such as button or cremini), chopped

4 thyme sprigs, leaves picked and chopped

3½ cups Chicken Bone Broth (page 146), plus extra if desired

3 slices bacon

Sea salt and freshly ground black pepper

1 handful watercress

Drizzle of extra-virgin olive oil

NUTRITION INFORMATION: Calories 747.7 | 38.5g total fat (18.9g saturated fat, 0.3g trans fat) | 1408.8mg cholesterol | 985mg sodium | 19.5g total carbohydrate (3.4g dietary fiber, 6.9g total sugars, 0g added sugars) | 79.3g protein | 0.2mcg vitamin D | 94.5mg calcium | 31mg iron | 1299.9mg potassium

FIRE TONIC

This is a powerful combination of warming, digestive-stimulating herbs in a base of unpasteurized apple cider vinegar. Unlike other fire tonic recipes, this one does not contain any chiles, which can be irritating to the gut.

Serves: 12 to 15

2 cups apple cider vinegar, plus extra if needed

10 garlic cloves, roughly chopped

4 ounces fresh horseradish, roughly chopped

4 ounces ginger, roughly chopped

1 celery stalk, chopped

1 carrot, chopped

1 onion, chopped

1-inch piece of fresh turmeric, chopped, or 1 teaspoon ground turmeric

1 tablespoon mustard seeds

a few flat-leaf parsley stalks, roughly chopped

a few rosemary sprigs, roughly chopped

a few oregano sprigs, roughly chopped

a few thyme sprigs, roughly chopped

1 tablespoon juniper berries

1 tablespoon black peppercorns

3 fresh bay leaves

1 tablespoon licorice root sticks

1 teaspoon sea salt

1. You will need a half-gallon preserving jar with an airtight lid for this recipe. Wash the jar and the utensils you plan to use thoroughly in very hot, soapy water, then run them through the dishwasher on a hot rinse cycle to sterilize. Alternatively, place them in a large saucepan filled with water and boil for 10 minutes, then place them on a baking tray in a 300 °F oven to dry.

2. Place all the ingredients in a glass or stainless steel bowl and mix well. Fill the jar with the vegetable and herb mix, pressing down firmly with a large spoon or potato masher to remove any air pockets. The vegetables and herbs should be completely submerged in the liquid, so add more vinegar if necessary.

3. Add a small glass weight (a shot glass is ideal) to keep everything submerged. Close the lid, then wrap a tea towel around the jar to block out the light.

4. Store the jar in a dark place with a temperature of 60 to 75 °F for 14 days. (You can place the jar in a small cooler to maintain a consistent temperature.)

5. Strain the tonic into a clean jar with a lid. Discard the vegetables, herbs, and spices.

6. Chill the fire tonic before serving. Keeps in the refrigerator, in a sealed glass jar, for 6 to 9 months.

NUTRITION INFORMATION: Calories 48.1 | 0.8g total fat (0.1g saturated fat, 0g trans fat) | 0mg cholesterol | 461.7mg sodium | 10.4g total carbohydrate (2.3g dietary fiber, 1.9g total sugars, 0g added sugars) | 1.1g protein | 0mcg vitamin D | 53.9mg calcium | 1.6mg iron | 134.2mg potassium

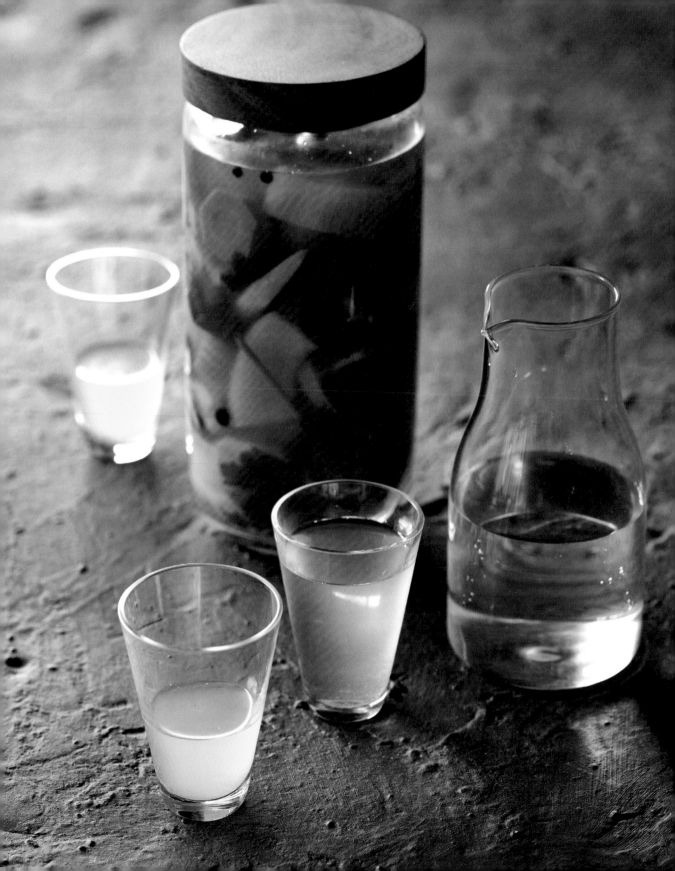

GARLIC AND HONEY TEA

I know what you may be thinking: Garlic . . . in tea? Yes! Boiling is a great way to extract the healing properties of garlic, and the lemon and honey keep its flavor from being overpowering. If you've ever heard the advice to eat a raw clove of garlic to keep viruses at bay, this tea enables you to enjoy garlic's protection without having to endure either the spicy bite of raw garlic or the challenge of swallowing it whole.

Serves: 2 to 3

4 cups filtered water

**2 garlic bulbs,
cut in half horizontally**

2 lemons, halved

¼ cup manuka or raw honey

1. Place the water, garlic, and lemons in a saucepan, bring to a boil over medium heat, then turn down to low and gently simmer for 1 hour so the flavors can develop.

2. Mix in the honey and allow to steep for 30 minutes.

3. When you're ready to drink the tea, reheat it until warmed through. Strain into cups or mugs and serve.

Any remaining tea will keep in a covered glass jar in the refrigerator for up to 1 week.

NUTRITION INFORMATION: Calories 334.1 | 0.5g total fat (0.1g saturated fat, 0g trans fat) | 0mg cholesterol | 23.8mg sodium | 78.9g total carbohydrate (4.7g dietary fiber, 56.9g total sugars, 0g added sugars) | 7.8g protein | 0mcg vitamin D | 60.2mg calcium | 2.5mg iron | 666.8mg potassium

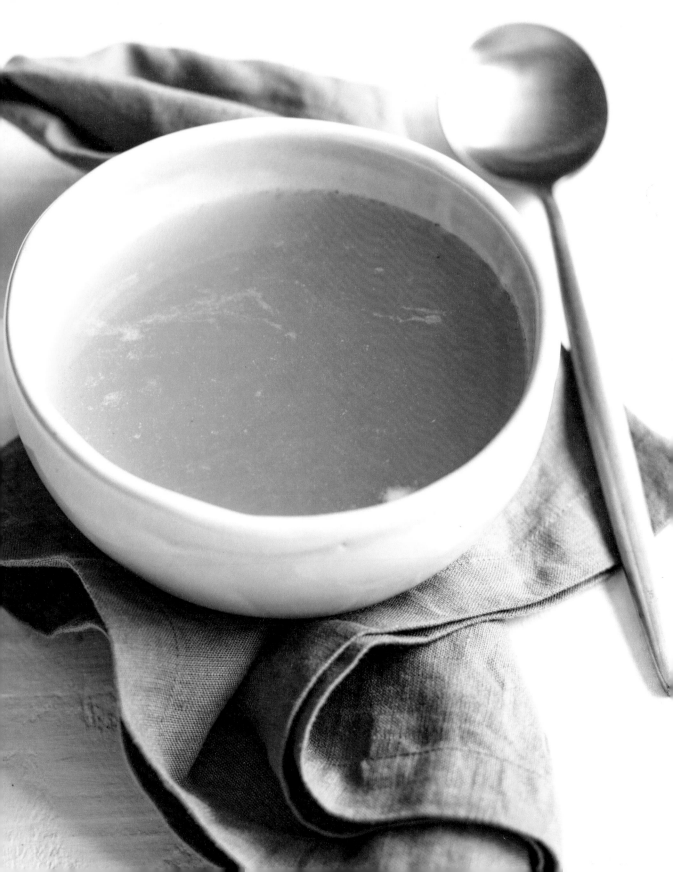

GINGER

- Overall digestive tonic

- Powerful anti-inflammatory

- Shown to be effective in treating a wide range of conditions and diseases, from asthma, autoimmunity, cancer, diabetes, heart disease, and more

Refer to page 21 for more information.

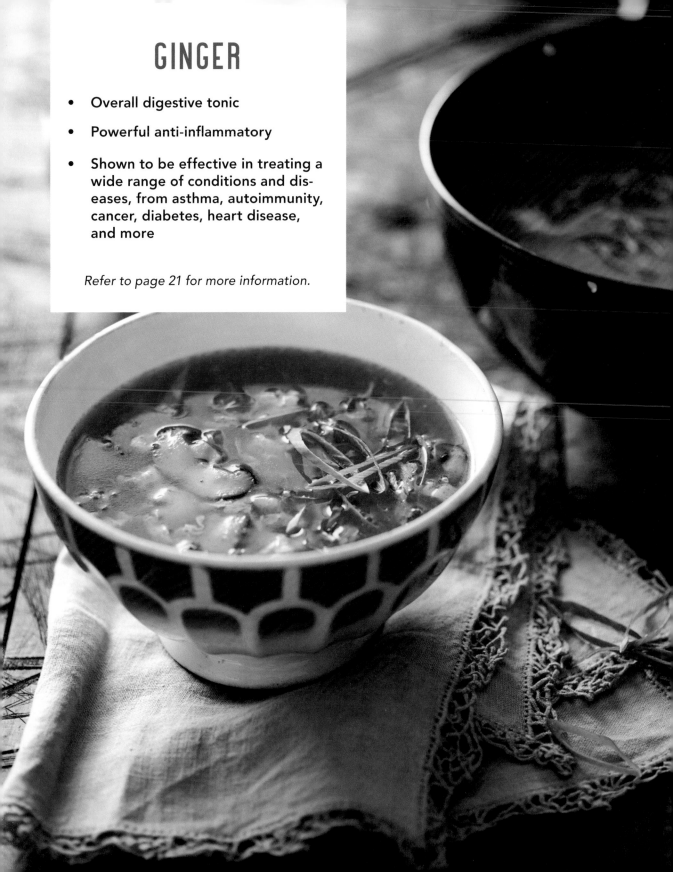

HOT-AND-SOUR SOUP

This staple of Chinese cuisine is as delicious as it is restorative. You'll love being able to re-create it at home. The fresh grated ginger makes it an anti-inflammatory and spicy treat.

1. Mix the tamari, vinegar, sesame oil, and honey in a bowl and set aside.

2. Heat the oil in a large saucepan over medium-high heat. Add the shallot, ginger, cilantro root, and chile and cook for 2 minutes or until the shallot and chile have softened and the mixture is fragrant.

3. Add the wood ear and shiitake mushrooms, bamboo shoots, kaffir lime leaves, and about half of the stock and simmer for 10 minutes. Stir in the tamari mixture.

4. Mix the tapioca flour with the remaining stock and stir into the soup. Continue to simmer until the soup thickens slightly, about 3 minutes.

5. Slowly pour the whisked eggs into the soup in a steady stream while gently stirring. Simmer for 30 seconds or until the eggs are cooked and look stringy. Add salt to taste, and if you prefer your soup to be quite sour, add a little more vinegar. Ladle the soup into serving bowls and garnish with the spring onion.

NOTE: Brown and ear shaped, wood ear mushrooms are commonly used in Chinese cuisine. They are available from Asian grocers.

Serves: 6

4 tablespoons tamari or coconut aminos

3 tablespoons apple cider vinegar

1 tablespoon toasted sesame oil

1 teaspoon honey

1 tablespoon coconut oil or other good-quality fat

2 shallots, finely diced

1½-inch piece ginger, peeled and grated

1 teaspoon finely chopped cilantro root (or the stems if your market doesn't sell cilantro with the roots attached)

1 long red chile, seeded and chopped

12 fresh wood ear mushrooms (about 1½ ounces), sliced (see note)

4 fresh shiitake mushrooms (about 2 ounces), sliced

½ cup bamboo shoots, sliced

2 kaffir lime leaves, torn

8 cups chicken stock

2½ tablespoons tapioca flour

3 eggs, whisked

Sea salt

1 spring onion, thinly sliced on the diagonal

NUTRITION INFORMATION: Calories 183.2 | 9.5g total fat (2.9g saturated fat, 0.1g trans fat) | 85.5mg cholesterol | 1189.3mg sodium | 10.4g total carbohydrate (1.2g dietary fiber, 2.7g total sugars, 1g added sugars) | 12.6g protein | 0.6mcg vitamin D | 66.8mg calcium | 1.7mg iron | 467.6mg potassium

GREEN JUICE with GINGER and LIME

Green juices are, of course, so much better for you than a soft drink or energy drink, as you can get a whole heap of nutrients in a single glass. On the downside, however, you are missing out on all of the amazing fiber in the veggies by juicing them. Another important thing to note is that, unlike a smoothie, a green juice will never be able to replace a meal because it doesn't have enough protein and fiber to keep you full. So if you are juicing in the morning, include some healthy dietary fat in your breakfast to make sure you won't be starving by 9 A.M.

Serves: 2

2½ bunches watercress (about ½ pound)

4 celery stalks

2 mini cucumbers (also called Lebanese cucumbers)

1 lime, peeled

2 handfuls flat-leaf parsley leaves

1 handful mint leaves

4-inch piece ginger

1 green apple, cored and chopped

1 tablespoon green superfood powder (optional; see note)

1. Combine all the ingredients except the superfood powder (if using) in a juicer and juice together.

2. Stir in the superfood powder.

3. Pour into two tall glasses and serve immediately.

NOTE: Green superfood powders contain a blend of powdered algae and green vegetables, providing a concentrated hit of antioxidants, vitamins, and minerals. They are available from health food stores and pharmacies.

NUTRITION INFORMATION: Calories 365.6 | 10.8g total fat (0.8g saturated fat, 0g trans fat) | 0mg cholesterol | 689.3mg sodium | 65.2g total carbohydrate (18.9g dietary fiber, 18.5g total sugars, 0g added sugars) | 19g protein | 0mcg vitamin D | 122.2mg calcium | 0.9mg iron | 623mg potassium

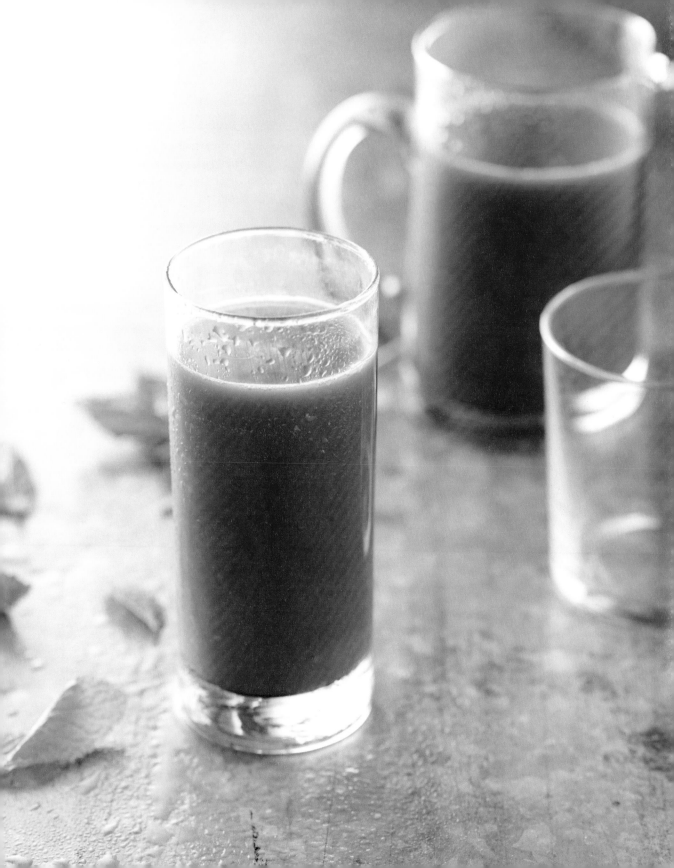

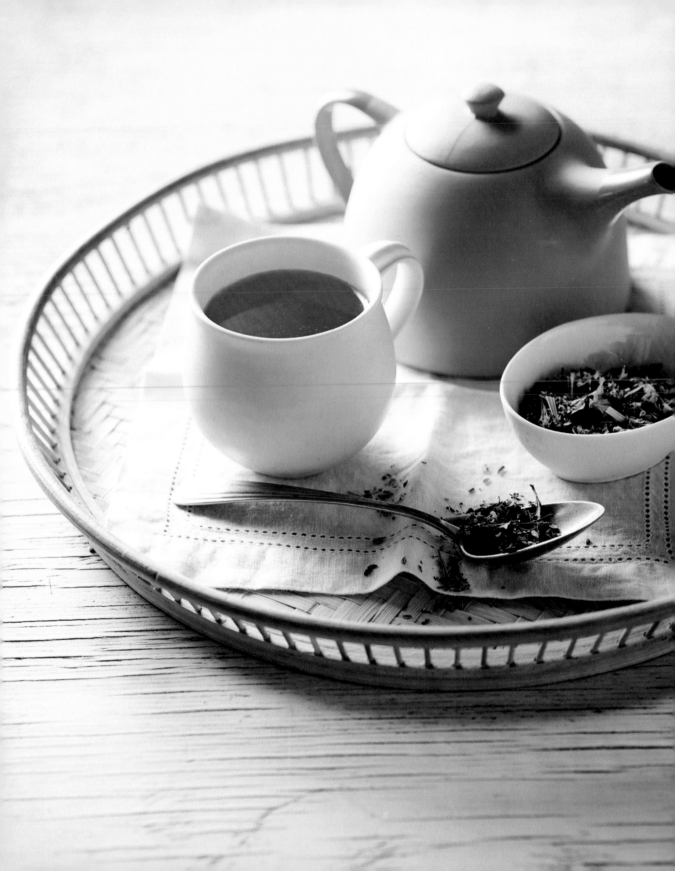

GUT-SOOTHING TEA

Just as the name suggests, this tea is like a gentle hug for your gut. All of the ingredients have wonderful anti-inflammatory properties: Licorice and slippery elm are both demulcent herbs that soothe an inflamed gut wall, calendula helps heal it by increasing the proliferation of cells required for wound repair, lemon balm calms the central nervous system, and lemongrass and ginger provide anti-inflammatory effects while stimulating circulation.

1. Mix all the ingredients in a bowl to combine. Place in an airtight container and store in a cupboard for up to 3 months.

2. For each cup of tea, steep 1 heaping teaspoon of the dried herb mixture in 1 cup of boiling water until cool enough to drink.

3. Sip slowly.

NOTE: You can buy dried calendula flowers, lemongrass tea, and ginger tea from health food stores or online. (We like the Southern Light Herbs brand.) Feel free to replace the lemongrass tea and ginger tea with the same amount of finely chopped lemongrass and finely grated ginger. Just add these fresh ingredients to each brew (you can prepare them in advance and store them in the freezer).

Serves: 8

1 teaspoon slippery elm powder

1 tablespoon licorice root sticks

1 tablespoon dried calendula flowers or calendula tea leaves (see note)

1 tablespoon dried lemon balm leaves

1 tablespoon lemongrass tea leaves (see note)

1 tablespoon ginger tea leaves (see note)

NUTRITION INFORMATION: Nutrition information for this recipe is not readily available

TULSI JELLIES

Tulsi, or holy basil, is known in India as the queen of herbs—and for good reason. It is full of antioxidants and is believed to promote well-being. Drinking the tea of this healing herb is said to boost the immune system; support liver function, which is essential for digestive health; and relieve stress. I recommend having a pot of tulsi tea every day and making these delicious jellies to enjoy as treats.

Makes: 30 servings

2½ tablespoons powdered gelatin

3 tablespoons tulsi tea leaves (see note)

1-inch piece ginger, sliced

2 tablespoons honey (optional)

Pinch sea salt

1. Place the gelatin in a small bowl. Pour 4 tablespoons of water over it and set aside to soak for 5 minutes or until the gelatin granules soften and expand.

2. Place the tulsi tea leaves and ginger in a large, heat-proof bowl and pour in 2 cups of boiling water. Whisk in the softened gelatin, cover with plastic wrap, and allow to steep for 30 minutes.

3. Strain the mixture into a jar.

4. Stir in the honey (if using) and salt. Pour into silicone molds and place in the fridge until set, about 4 hours. Store the jellies in an airtight container in the fridge for up to 2 weeks.

NOTE: You can find tulsi tea leaves at health food stores and some supermarkets.

NUTRITION INFORMATION: Calories 250.5 | 0.1g total fat (0g saturated fat, 0g trans fat) | 0mg cholesterol | 216mg sodium | 35.9g total carbohydrate (0.2g dietary fiber, 34.9g total sugars, 34.8g added sugars) | 30.2g protein | 0mcg vitamin D | 23mg calcium | 0.6mg iron | 50.5mg potassium

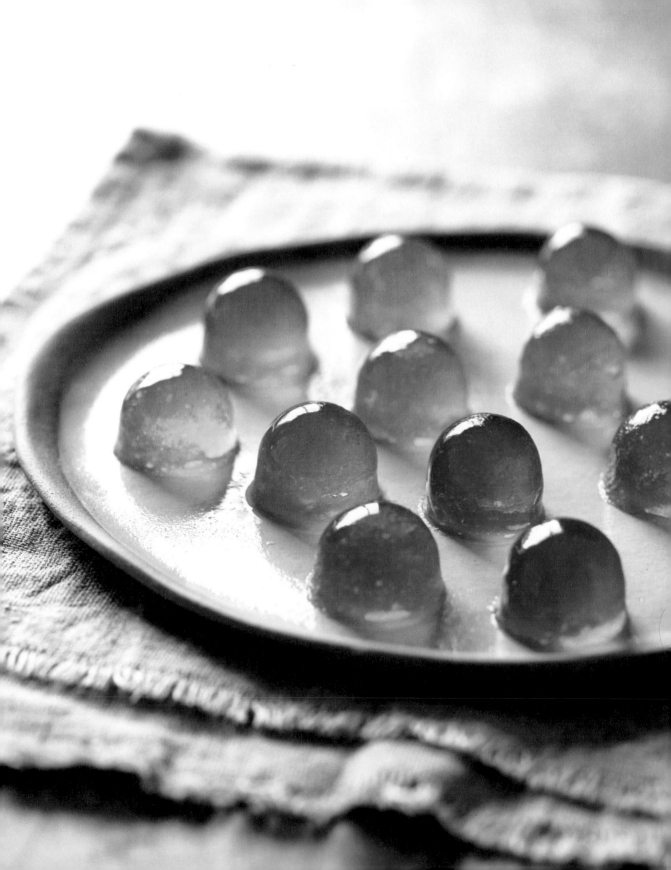

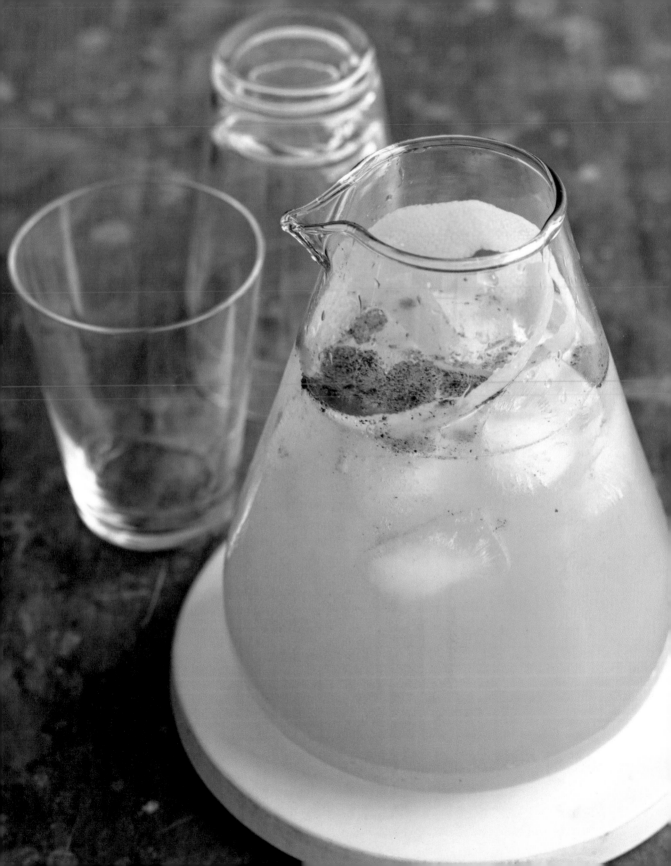

CLOVE AND GINGER LEMONADE ELIXIR

Drink this tea on an empty stomach in the morning to stimulate digestion and detoxification. The lemon is alkalinizing, the ginger is warming and soothing to your stomach, and the cinnamon will help regulate your blood sugar. After a cup of this, you'll be ready for anything!

1. Place all ingredients in a medium saucepan and bring to a gentle simmer, stirring until the honey has dissolved.

2. Remove from heat, cover with a lid, and allow to steep for 1 hour so the spices and ginger can infuse.

3. Strain through a fine sieve into a jar and discard the spices and ginger. Refrigerate until chilled. Sprinkle with an extra pinch of ground clove and serve with ice.

Serves: 4

¾ cup plus 1 tablespoon lemon juice

4 cups filtered water

1¼-inch piece ginger, sliced

1 pinch ground clove, plus extra to serve

3 cardamom pods, crushed

1 cinnamon stick

½ cup manuka honey or maple syrup, or any sweetener of your choice (add to taste)

NUTRITION INFORMATION: Calories 73.7 | 0.2g total fat (0g saturated fat, 0g trans fat) | 0mg cholesterol | 2.1mg sodium | 18.4g total carbohydrate (1.8g dietary fiber, 12.8g total sugars, 0g added sugars) | 1g protein | 0mcg vitamin D | 26mg calcium | 0.8mg iron | 129.8mg potassium

GINGER SWITCHEL

If you haven't heard of switchel, basically it's one of the world's first soft drinks, made by adding apple cider vinegar, spices, and herbs to still or sparking water. It is a great alternative to kombucha or kefir as the apple cider vinegar is wonderful on the gut and has anti-inflammatory properties.

Serves: 4

4 cups coconut water

2 tablespoons apple cider vinegar

1 to 2 tablespoons monk fruit sweetener, maple syrup, or honey

1 tablespoon finely chopped ginger

1. You'll need a half-gallon mason jar with a lid for this recipe. Wash the jar in very hot water or run through a hot rinse cycle in the dishwasher.

2. Place all ingredients in the prepared jar and mix well.

3. Cover and refrigerate for 12 hours to infuse.

4. After 12 hours, strain the ginger switchel into glasses, add some ice, and serve.

NUTRITION INFORMATION: Calories 51.5 | 0.5g total fat (0.5g saturated fat, 0g trans fat) | 0mg cholesterol | 252.3mg sodium | 14.6g total carbohydrate (7.5g dietary fiber, 6.3g total sugars, 0g added sugars) | 1.8g protein | 0mcg vitamin D | 59.5mg calcium | 1mg iron | 621.7mg potassium

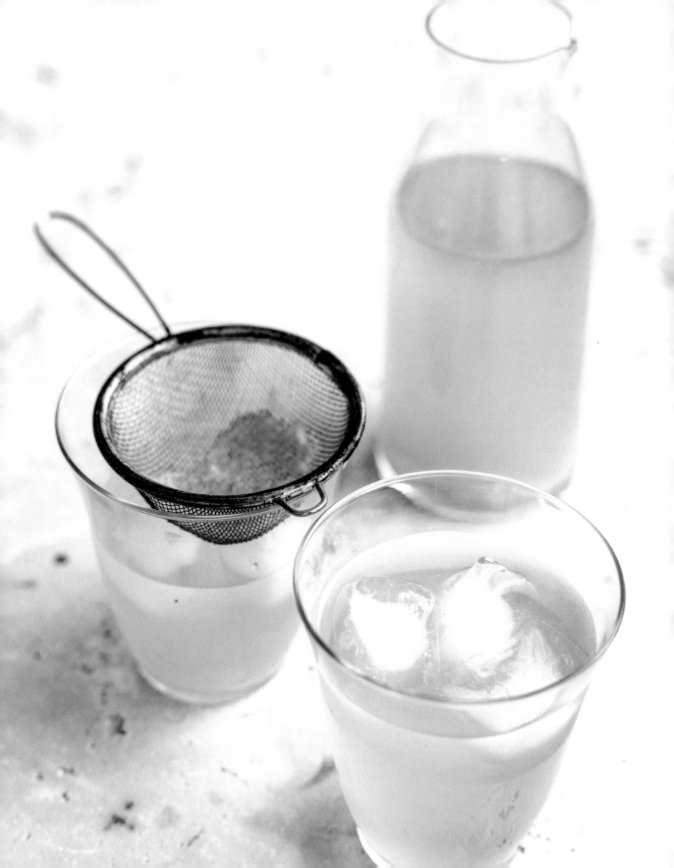

WARM COCONUT CHAI

This recipe comes from a friend whose warm coconut chai is nearly as famous as her tea ceremonies.

Chai, a wonderfully fragrant spiced tea that originated in India, is a very popular beverage all around the world, traditionally made with black tea leaves, cinnamon, cardamom, ginger, black pepper, and cloves. Here, to add a wonderful element of fat that will keep you satiated for longer, we have used coconut cream or coconut milk as the base. I encourage you to try this as a warming drink in the cooler months or enjoy it chilled or served over ice in summer.

Serves: 2 to 4

4 cinnamon sticks

16 cardamom pods, bruised

16 whole cloves

2-inch piece ginger, sliced

1 teaspoon black peppercorns

1 teaspoon fennel seeds

4 star anise

1 tablespoon tulsi tea leaves (caffeine-free)

3 tablespoons coconut cream or coconut milk, or more if desired

Honey or liquid stevia, to taste (optional)

1. Bring 3 cups of water to a boil in a saucepan.

2. Reduce the heat to low, add the spices and tea leaves, and gently simmer for 15 minutes to allow the flavors to develop.

3. Stir in the coconut cream or milk and bring to a simmer, then remove from the heat.

4. Strain the tea through a fine strainer into a heatproof jar or teapot, then pour into mugs.

5. Stir a little honey or stevia into the chai for a touch of sweetness, if desired.

NUTRITION INFORMATION: Calories 481.6 | 17.8g total fat (0.9g saturated fat, 0g trans fat) | 0mg cholesterol | 57.3mg sodium | 78.4g total carbohydrate (24.1g dietary fiber, 1.7g total sugars, 0g added sugars) | 31g protein | 0.1mcg vitamin D | 754.6mg calcium | 40.8mg iron | 401.8mg potassium

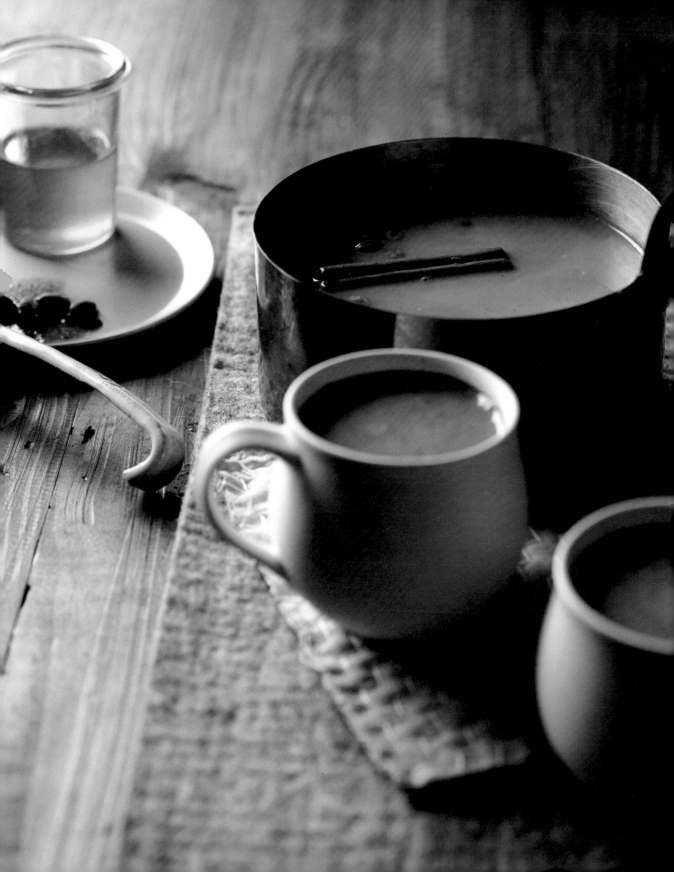

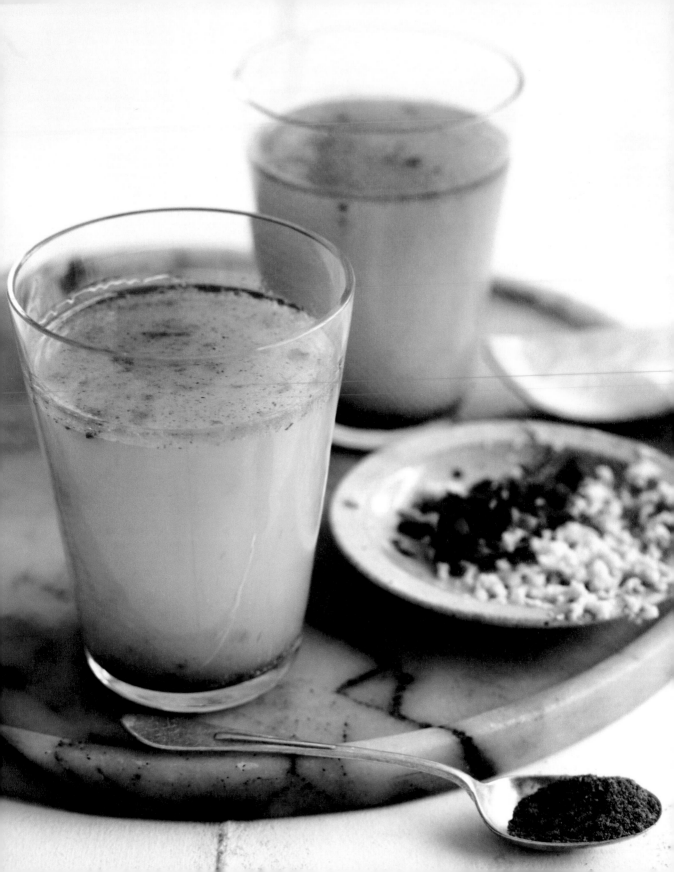

IMMUNE-BOOSTING CHICKEN BROTH
WITH A TON OF GOODNESS

I'd like to replace the old saying "An apple a day keeps the doctor away" with "A broth a day keeps the doctor away," especially if you include immune-boosting ingredients such as ginger, cayenne pepper, lemon juice, and parsley. You can make this recipe with different combinations of ingredients. Try adding some slippery elm, licorice root, and pau d'arco for gut support. Or throw in sliced medicinal mushrooms or truffles, bean sprouts, and herbs. Other combinations you might like include collagen, gelatin, and MCT oil; turmeric, garlic, and ashwagandha . . . the options are almost endless!

1. Place the broth in a saucepan and bring to a simmer over medium heat.

2. Add the ginger, cayenne pepper, and lemon juice and stir to combine.

3. Season with salt and pepper to taste.

4. Pour the hot broth into two mugs and sprinkle the chopped parsley on top.

Serves: 2

3 cups Chicken Bone Broth (page 146)

2 tablespoons finely grated ginger

¼ teaspoon cayenne pepper

2 teaspoons lemon juice, or to taste

Sea salt and freshly ground black pepper

1 tablespoon finely chopped flat-leaf parsley

NUTRITION INFORMATION: Calories 91.9 | 3.5g total fat (1.2g saturated fat, 0g trans fat) | 2.6mg cholesterol | 491.6mg sodium | 9.5g total carbohydrate (1.8g dietary fiber, 1.1g total sugars, 0g added sugars) | 6.4g protein | 0.1mcg vitamin D | 29.5mg calcium | 2.8mg iron | 382.2mg potassium

HEALING CHICKEN AND VEGETABLE SOUP

People around the world have known about the healing benefits of chicken soup for millennia. It is as powerful a medicine as ever—helping to heal the lining of your gut, boosting immunity, and contributing to the health of your joints. Just remember that it's essential to use homemade chicken bone broth in this recipe to get maximum nutritional benefit.

Serves: 6

One 3½-pound chicken

Chicken Bone Broth (page 146)

2 tablespoons coconut oil or other good-quality fat

1 onion, chopped

3 garlic cloves, crushed

1 large carrot, chopped

1 celery stalk, halved lengthwise and cut into ⅓-inch-thick slices

4 thyme sprigs

1 bay leaf

1 tablespoon finely grated ginger

1 large zucchini, halved lengthwise and sliced into ¾-inch-thick slices

1½ cups peeled and cubed butternut squash (¾-inch cubes)

1 cup Swiss chard, tough stems removed, sliced into ribbons

Sea salt and freshly ground black pepper

1 handful flat-leaf parsley leaves, finely chopped (optional)

1. First, heat a large pot full of Chicken Bone Broth to a simmer (leaving enough room in the pot to accommodate the chicken). Then submerge the whole chicken in the broth, adding some water if necessary to completely cover it.

2. Simmer, uncovered, for 1 hour, or until the chicken is cooked through.

3. Carefully remove the chicken from the broth and allow to cool slightly.

4. Meanwhile, follow the instructions for straining and skimming the broth on page 146.

5. When chicken is cool enough to handle, shred the flesh and discard the bones. Cover and refrigerate until needed.

6. Place a stockpot or very large saucepan over medium heat and coat the base with the oil or fat.

7. Add the onion, garlic, carrot, celery, thyme, and bay leaf and cook, stirring, for about 6 minutes or until the vegetables are soft but not browned. Pour in 3 cups of the poaching liquid and bring to a boil, then turn down to a simmer and cook for 20 minutes.

8. Add the ginger, zucchini, and butternut squash to the pot and continue to cook for a further 15 minutes, or until the vegetables are tender. Add about 2 cups of the shredded poached chicken and the chard and continue to simmer for another few minutes until the chard is cooked and the chicken is warmed through. Season to taste with salt and pepper, sprinkle with the parsley (if using), and serve.

NUTRITION INFORMATION: Calories 503.1 | 13.9g total fat (6.8g saturated fat, 0g trans fat) | 273.3mg cholesterol | 241.8mg sodium | 18.2g total carbohydrate (3.2g dietary fiber, 6.3g total sugars, 3.2g added sugars) | 83.3g protein | 0.1mcg vitamin D | 61.4mg calcium | 2.9mg iron | 1314.1mg potassium

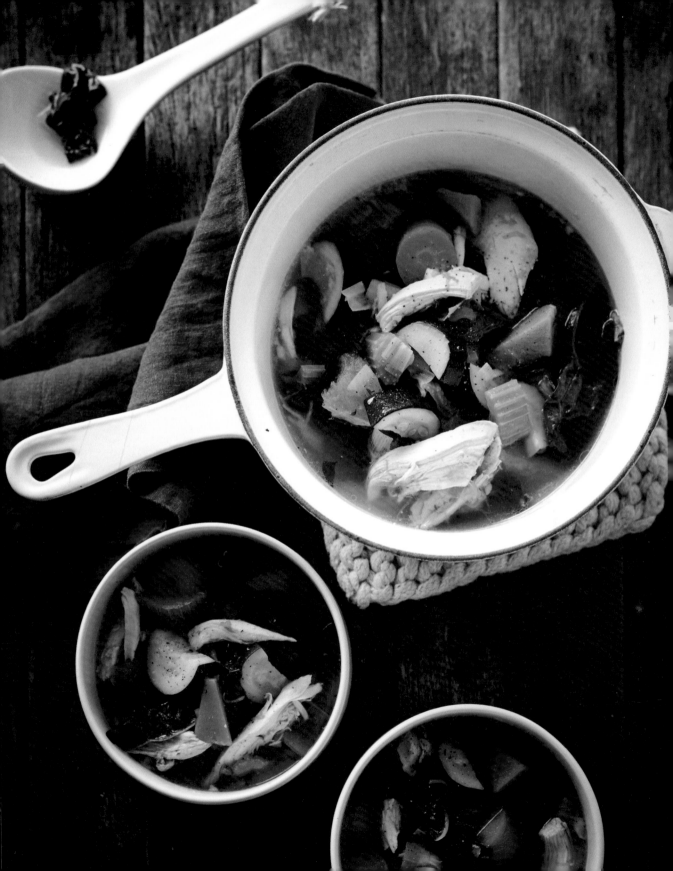

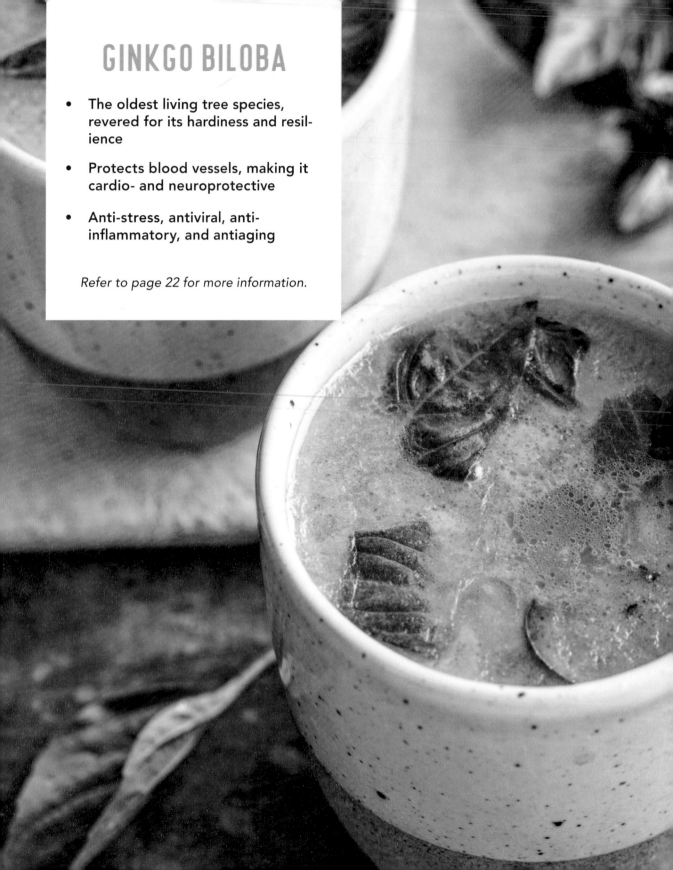

GINKGO BILOBA

- The oldest living tree species, revered for its hardiness and resilience

- Protects blood vessels, making it cardio- and neuroprotective

- Anti-stress, antiviral, anti-inflammatory, and antiaging

Refer to page 22 for more information.

GINKGO CHICKEN BROTH

In the United States, most people take their ginkgo in supplement form, but stirring it into homemade Chicken Bone Broth is much more delicious—and makes your bone broth that much more immunity boosting. Dried ginkgo leaves are available at Asian markets or online.

1. Place the bone broth in a medium saucepan, stir in the dried ginkgo leaves and fresh turmeric, cover with a lid, and bring to a boil.

2. As soon as the broth comes to the boil, remove it from the heat and allow it to steep for 1 hour. If not serving right away, store in the refrigerator in a glass container with a tightly fitting lid.

3. To serve, reheat the broth in a saucepan until it is hot, then stir in the lemon juice and holy basil. Season with sea salt and freshly cracked pepper to taste.

4. Pour into mugs and enjoy!

Serves: 4

4 cups Chicken Bone Broth (page 146)

2 tablespoons dried ginkgo leaves

1 teaspoon freshly grated turmeric

1 to 2 teaspoons lemon juice, or to taste

1 large handful holy basil (tulsi) leaves

Sea salt and freshly cracked pepper

NUTRITION INFORMATION: Nutrition information for this recipe is not readily available

KOREAN GINSENG, CHICKEN, AND CAULIFLOWER SOUP

You can almost feel this flavorful soup restoring you from the inside out. Red dates are among the most popular health foods in China, where they are hailed for their ability to rectify low energy, both diarrhea and constipation, and insomnia. They are available at Asian markets or online.

Serves: 6

1½ cups roughly chopped cauli-flower (florets and stalk)

6 garlic cloves, chopped

10 red dates (jujubes), halved

5 fresh or dried chestnuts, peeled and thinly sliced

3 fresh or dried ginseng roots, sliced lengthwise

One 4-pound chicken

12 cups Chicken Bone Broth (page 146)

2 tablespoons tamari

2 tablespoons finely grated ginger

Sea salt

2 spring onions, finely chopped

1 teaspoon sesame seeds, toasted

2 teaspoons sesame oil

1 to 2 teaspoons Korean red chili paste (gochujang) (optional)

1. Place the cauliflower in a food processor and pulse into tiny, fine pieces that look like rice.

2. Transfer the cauliflower rice to a large bowl, then add 2 chopped garlic cloves, 2 dates, 2 sliced chestnuts, and 1 sliced ginseng root and mix well.

3. Stuff the cavity of the chicken with the cauliflower mixture, making sure it is firmly filled. Tie the legs of the chicken together with kitchen string so the cauliflower doesn't escape.

4. Place the chicken, neck first, in a narrow and deep saucepan that holds it snugly. Add the remaining garlic, dates, chestnuts, and ginseng along with the broth, tamari, and ginger.

5. Bring the soup to a simmer over medium heat, skimming any scum that rises to the top. You don't want to boil the soup too vigorously. Cover the pan, reduce the heat, and simmer for 1 hour or until the chicken is cooked. Remove from the heat.

6. Remove and discard the string from the chicken, then scoop out the cauliflower rice from the chicken cavity and add to the soup, along with the spring onions and sesame oil.

7. Season with salt to taste.

8. Carefully remove the chicken from the pan and carve or shred into pieces. Place the chicken in a warm serving bowl, then ladle the soup on top.

NUTRITION INFORMATION: Calories 629.3 | 16.8g total fat (5.1g saturated fat, 0.1g trans fat) | 334.8mg cholesterol | 1252.7mg sodium | 9.7g total carbohydrate (1.6g dietary fiber, 3.2g total sugars, 0.1g added sugars) | 109.8g protein | 0.2mcg vitamin D | 56.8mg calcium | 3.4mg iron | 1927.8mg potassium

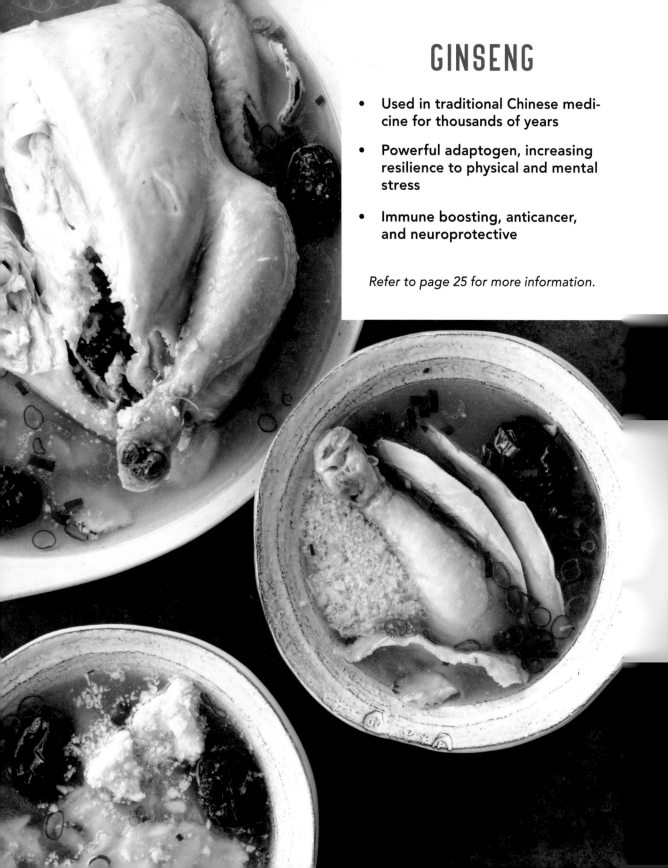

GINSENG

- Used in traditional Chinese medicine for thousands of years

- Powerful adaptogen, increasing resilience to physical and mental stress

- Immune boosting, anticancer, and neuroprotective

Refer to page 25 for more information.

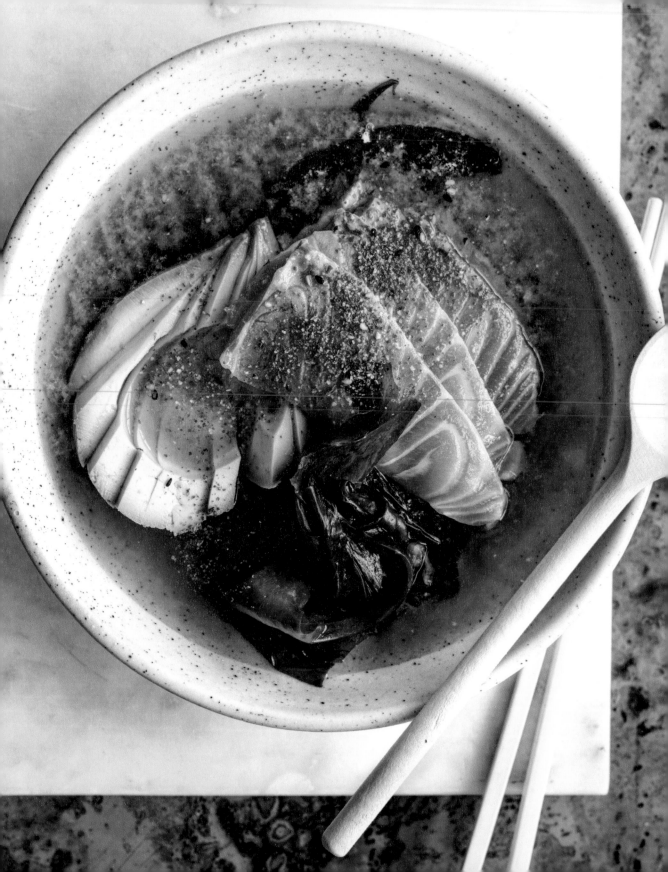

SEAWEED SOUP WITH SALMON, AVOCADO, AND GINSENG

If you could serve good health in a bowl, it would be this soup. The kombu and wakame (both types of seaweed) are chock-full of trace minerals and are also a great source of fiber and protein. In addition, the ginseng delivers an immunity boost, the miso brings flavor (and probiotics for gut health), and the salmon and avocado make this tasty soup a delivery system for healthy fats. There are some ingredients that might be unfamiliar to home cooks: dashi powder is a concentrated form of a savory broth that is a staple in Japanese cooking; miso is fermented soybean paste with a wonderful salty flavor, and shichimi togarashi is a Japanese seven-spice blend that lends a little heat. They are all available in Asian markets and make healthful and tasty additions to your cooking repertoire.

NOTE: You'll need to start this recipe a day ahead.

1. To start on the broth, place the kombu, ginseng, and water or broth in a large, heavy-based saucepan. Cover and place in the fridge for at least 8 hours or overnight to allow the kombu and ginseng to soak.

2. The next day, place the pan over medium-high heat and bring to a simmer (do not boil). Reduce the heat to low and simmer for 15 minutes.

3. Add the dashi and continue to simmer for 5 minutes, then remove from the heat and allow to steep for 15 minutes. Remove and discard the kombu.

4. Soak the wakame in 1 cup of water for 5 minutes or until the wakame expands, then drain. If you like smaller pieces of seaweed in your miso soup, chop the wakame to your liking.

5. Whisk the miso into the broth and bring it back to a simmer. Add the wakame and simmer for 2 minutes, or until it is heated through.

6. Ladle the seaweed broth into soup bowls.

7. Add the raw salmon and avocado, sprinkle on the shichimi togarashi (if using), and serve.

Serves: 4

Two 4-inch sheets dried kombu

3 slices ginseng (each about 2 inches long)

6 cups water, fish broth, or Chicken Bone Broth (page 146)

2 teaspoons dashi powder

7 ounces dried wakame

⅓ cup white (shiro) miso paste

1 pound sashimi-grade salmon, skinned and cut into ¼-inch-thick slices

2 avocados, sliced

1 teaspoon shichimi togarashi, or to taste (optional)

NUTRITION INFORMATION: Calories 346.4 | 21.6g total fat (6.1g saturated fat, 0g trans fat) | 52.9mg cholesterol | 1735.1mg sodium | 12.8g total carbohydrate (5.5g dietary fiber, 0.7g total sugars, 0g added sugars) | 25.3g protein | 6.1mcg vitamin D | 34.1mg calcium | 1.4mg iron | 895.2mg potassium

GREEN TEA

I can think of no better daily morning ritual than to have a steaming cup of green tea. Adding mint leaves makes it smell as good as it tastes.

Serves: 2

1 tablespoon dried green tea leaves

1 handful fresh mint leaves, to serve

Manuka honey, to serve (optional)

1. Place the dried tea leaves in a teapot or jar, pour in 2 cups of boiling water, and allow to steep for 5 minutes.

2. Strain into cups and stir in the mint leaves. Add some manuka honey (if using), then slowly sip to enjoy.

NUTRITION INFORMATION: Calories 41.3 | 0g total fat (0g saturated fat, 0g trans fat) | 0mg cholesterol | 0.5mg sodium | 7.3g total carbohydrate (2.2g dietary fiber, 5g total sugars, 0g added sugars) | 2.1g protein | 0mcg vitamin D | 40mg calcium | 0.8mg iron | 9mg potassium

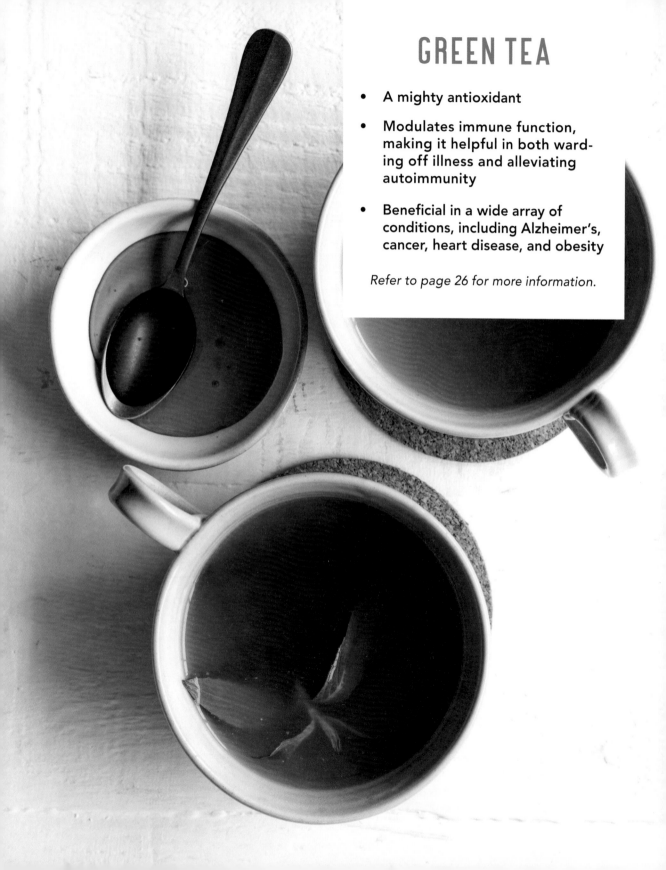

GREEN TEA

- A mighty antioxidant

- Modulates immune function, making it helpful in both warding off illness and alleviating autoimmunity

- Beneficial in a wide array of conditions, including Alzheimer's, cancer, heart disease, and obesity

Refer to page 26 for more information.

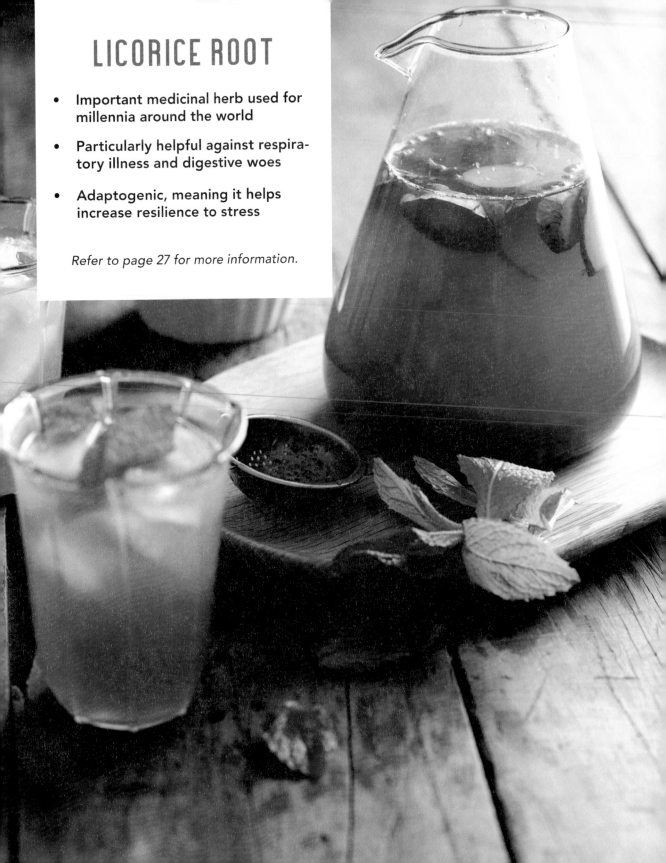

LICORICE ROOT

- Important medicinal herb used for millennia around the world

- Particularly helpful against respiratory illness and digestive woes

- Adaptogenic, meaning it helps increase resilience to stress

Refer to page 27 for more information.

GINGER AND LICORICE ICED TEA

I don't drink coffee, as it is a stimulant that can mess with your adrenal system. Anything that stimulates you is also likely to make you crash later, which means you feel the need for something else to pick you up again. Skipping coffee doesn't mean you have to miss out on pick-me-ups altogether, though. This licorice and ginger iced tea is an amazing way to begin your day—ginger is fabulous for digestion, and the licorice gives the drink a slightly sweet flavor, without actually being full of sugar. You can also experiment with different spice mixes in this tea; you could even jar them up and give them to friends and family as a gift.

1. Put the licorice root, ginger, and cinnamon in a large teapot and pour in 4 cups of boiling water. Allow to steep for 20 minutes.

2. Pour the tea through a fine strainer into a jar, then add the mint. Add the lemon (if using) and stir.

3. Of course, the tea can be enjoyed hot too. If you like, drink right away. If you're in the mood for iced tea, let cool to room temperature, then cover and chill in the refrigerator.

4. Strain and serve with ice cubes.

Serves: 2 to 4

4 tablespoons broken-up licorice root sticks

¾-inch piece ginger, sliced or grated

1 cinnamon stick

1 small handful mint leaves

Juice of 1 lemon (optional)

Ice cubes

NUTRITION INFORMATION: Calories 73.7 | 0.3g total fat (0.2g saturated fat, 0g trans fat) | 0mg cholesterol | 136.6mg sodium | 17.2g total carbohydrate (7g dietary fiber, 4g total sugars, 0g added sugars) | 2g protein | 0mcg vitamin D | 171.1mg calcium | 0.4mg iron | 58.2mg potassium

CHAMOMILE AND LICORICE TEA

A super-simple soothing tea for the gut and central nervous system. Chamomile is anti-inflammatory and great for easing digestive cramps and spasms. It also very gently stimulates digestion. Licorice is anti-inflammatory and demulcent, making it extra soothing for the gut.

Serves: 2

2 tablespoons dried chamomile flowers

1 tablespoon broken-up licorice root sticks

1. Fill two mugs with boiling water.

2. Evenly divide the chamomile flowers and licorice root between the mugs, stir, and leave to infuse for 3 minutes.

3. Strain and serve.

NUTRITION INFORMATION: Calories 76.5 | 0.1g total fat (0.1g saturated fat, 0g trans fat) | 0mg cholesterol | 85.5mg sodium | 7.8g total carbohydrate (3.1g dietary fiber, 2.2g total sugars, 0g added sugars) | 1.1g protein | 0mcg vitamin D | 85.2mg calcium | 0mg iron | 0mg potassium

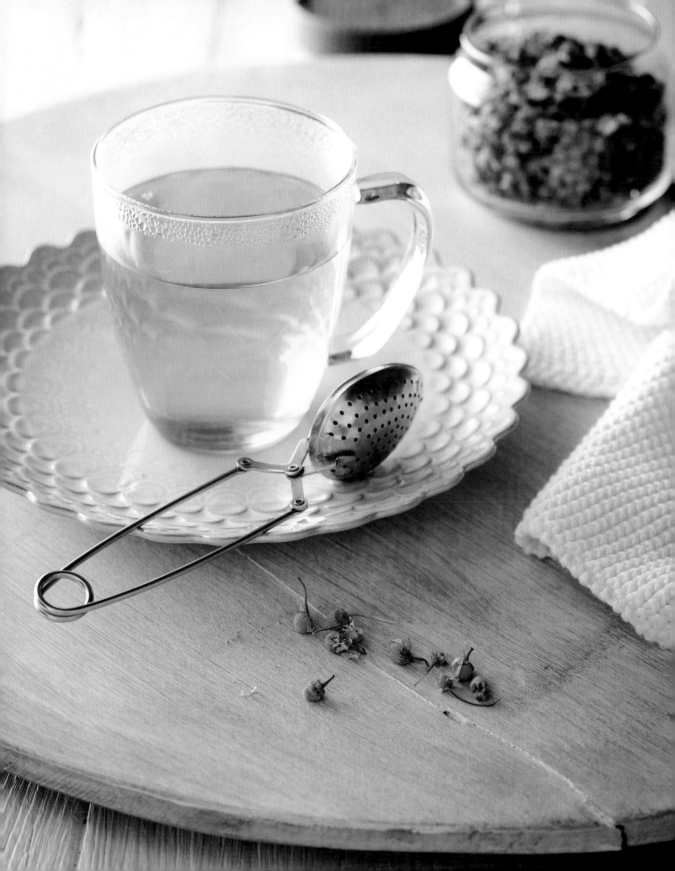

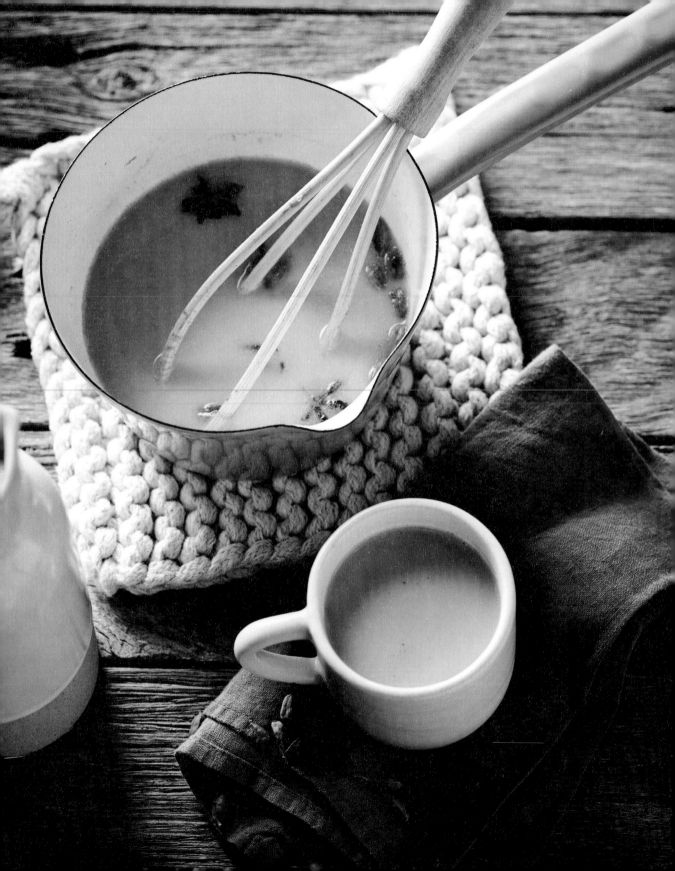

CHAI-BIOTIC

Chai-biotic means tea (chai) for life (biotic). This absolutely delicious warming and comforting tea is fantastic for helping to keep your gut and immune system in good shape. It's particularly great if you are experiencing any yeast problems, as the spices used are strong antifungals. They also stimulate blood circulation, which is wonderful if your fingers and toes are a bit cold or if your brain is a bit foggy.

1. Place the pau d'arco, cat's claw, and spices in a saucepan, add 1 cup of filtered water, bring to a simmer, and simmer for 5 minutes.

2. Add almond milk and strain through a sieve. Serve and savor.

NOTE: Leave out the cat's claw if you are pregnant or planning to become pregnant in the next two months. Cat's claw has traditionally been used as a contraceptive, and while there is no conclusive evidence as to its effectiveness, it is best to play it safe.

Serves: 1

1 teaspoon pau d'arco powder

1 teaspoon cat's claw powder (see note)

1 teaspoon ground cinnamon

½ teaspoon freshly grated nutmeg

3 cardamom pods or ¼ teaspoon ground cardamom

1 or 2 star anise

¼ teaspoon licorice root powder

¼ teaspoon ground turmeric

1 cup almond milk or coconut milk

NUTRITION INFORMATION: Calories 369.7 | 18.6g total fat (2.9g saturated fat, 0g trans fat) | 0mg cholesterol | 29.1mg sodium | 53.2g total carbohydrate (16.3g dietary fiber, 0.5g total sugars, 0g added sugars) | 18.5g protein | 1.6mcg vitamin D | 727.7mg calcium | 37.7mg iron | 52.3mg potassium

MY FAVORITE TEA

I love to sip a big cup of this tea after dinner—or at any time of day for that matter. Cloves are among the best antioxidants, and they don't cost a fortune. Ginger and licorice root are both wonderful digestive aids, making this cup of goodness an ideal after-dinner treat.

Serves: 2

1 teaspoon ground cinnamon

½ teaspoon ground cardamom

½ teaspoon ground cloves

1 teaspoon finely grated ginger

1 tablespoon licorice root powder

1 teaspoon honey

Coconut cream or coconut milk, to taste

1. Bring 4 cups of water to a boil in a saucepan.

2. Remove the pan from the heat. Add the cinnamon, cardamom, cloves, ginger, licorice root, and honey and allow to steep for 5 minutes.

3. Add the coconut cream, stir, and serve.

NUTRITION INFORMATION: Calories 33.2 | 0.3g total fat (0.2g saturated fat, 0g trans fat) | 0mg cholesterol | 57.6mg sodium | 7.4g total carbohydrate (3.2g dietary fiber, 1.5g total sugars, 0g added sugars) | 0.9g protein | 0mcg vitamin D | 75.6mg calcium | 0.4mg iron | 28.7mg potassium

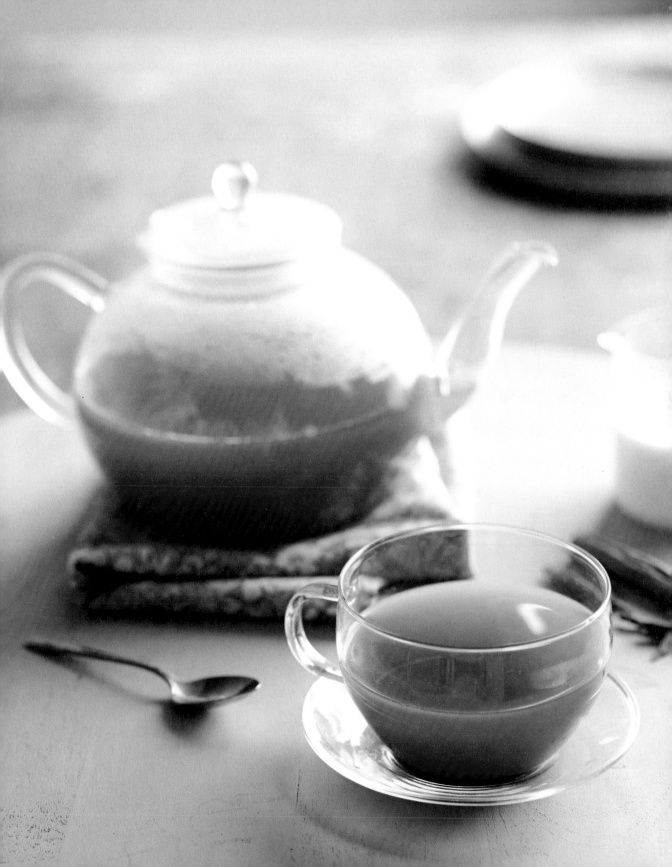

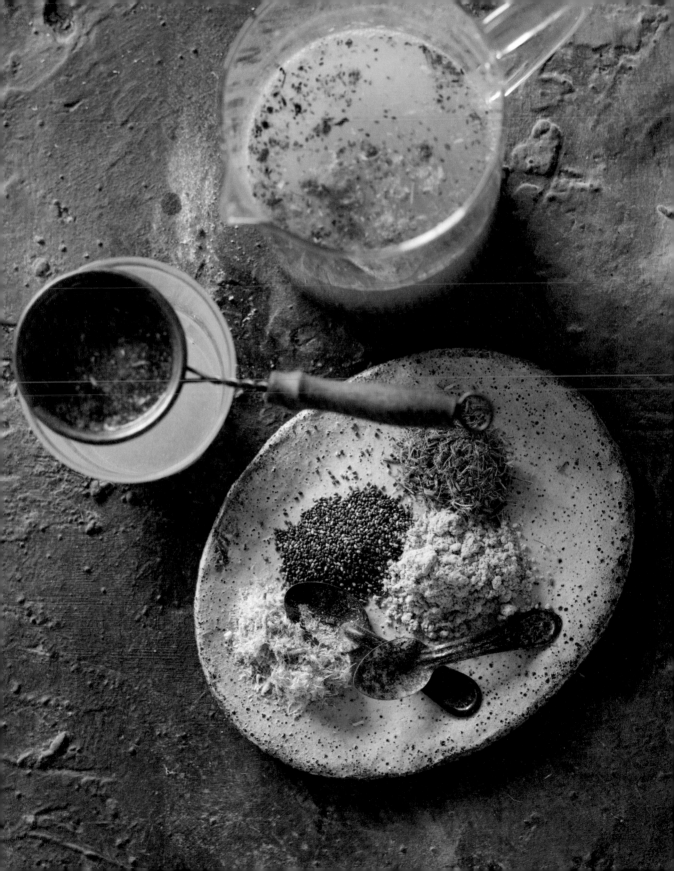

TONIC TEA

This satisfying, silky, and somewhat sweet tea is wonderfully soothing for the lining of your gut. Licorice, marshmallow root, chia seeds, and slippery elm have anti-inflammatory properties, while lemon helps to improve water absorption, stimulate the liver, and improve digestion. The gentle sweetness of licorice and cinnamon can help put any sweet cravings at bay, as well as help regulate insulin levels if you are adjusting to a low-carb diet.

1. Place the licorice and marshmallow root in a teapot or jar and pour in the boiling water. Allow to steep and cool for 15 minutes.

2. While the tea is steeping, place the cold water, chia seeds, cinnamon, slippery elm, and lemon juice in a blender.

3. Blend on high speed until smooth. Pour through a fine strainer into a jar.

4. Strain the steeped tea into the chia and cinnamon mixture. Stir, taste, and add more lemon juice if needed.

5. Chill the tea before drinking, or serve over ice, if you prefer. You can also drink it warm.

Serves: 4

2 tablespoons broken-up licorice root sticks

1 teaspoon marshmallow root

2 cups boiling filtered water

2 cups cold filtered water

½ teaspoon chia seeds

1 teaspoon ground cinnamon

½ teaspoon slippery elm powder

2 teaspoons lemon juice, plus extra if needed

Ice cubes (optional)

NUTRITION INFORMATION: Calories 29.9 | 0.2g total fat (0.1g saturated fat, 0g trans fat) | 0mg cholesterol | 59.6mg sodium | 6.3g total carbohydrate (2.7g dietary fiber, 1.6g total sugars, 0g added sugars) | 0.9g protein | 0mcg vitamin D | 68.5mg calcium | 0.1mg iron | 6mg potassium

OLIVE LEAF AND LEMON BALM TEA

Olive leaf is a powerful antiviral, and lemon balm is calming both to your nerves and to your digestive system, making this the perfect thing to drink when work gets busy or life gets stressful (which is when we tend to be more susceptible to infection).

Serves: 2

1 tablespoon dried olive leaves

2 teaspoons dried lemon balm leaves

1. Place the dried leaves into a teapot or jar, pour in 2 cups of boiling water, and allow to steep for 5 minutes.

2. Strain into cups and slowly sip to enjoy.

NUTRITION INFORMATION: Calories 185 | 0.6g total fat (0g saturated fat, 0g trans fat) | 0mg cholesterol | 0mg sodium | 43.8g total carbohydrate (0g dietary fiber, 0g total sugars, 0g added sugars) | 0.7g protein | 0mcg vitamin D | 0mg calcium | 0mg iron | 0mg potassium

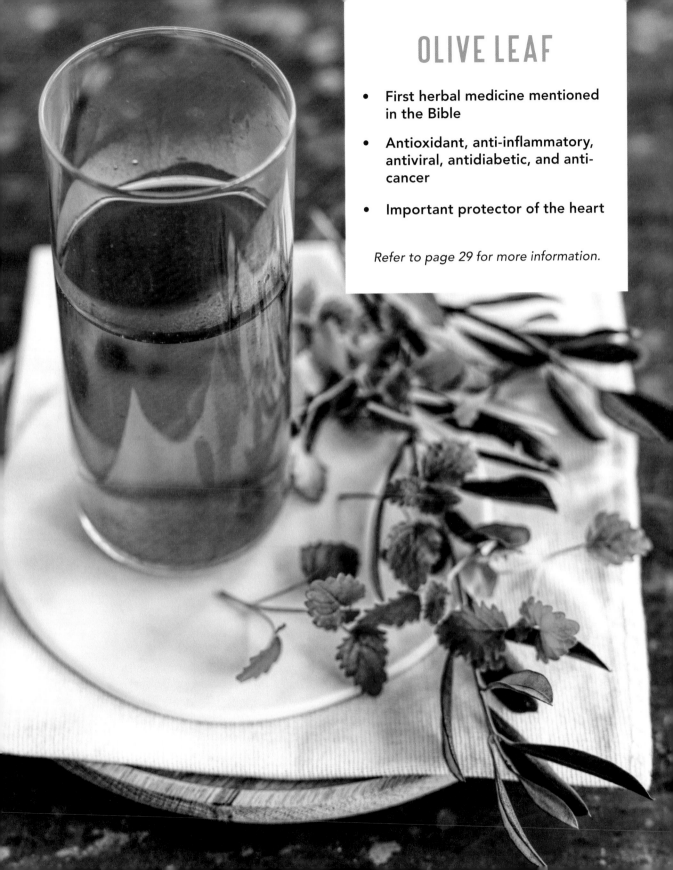

OLIVE LEAF

- First herbal medicine mentioned in the Bible

- Antioxidant, anti-inflammatory, antiviral, antidiabetic, and anti-cancer

- Important protector of the heart

Refer to page 29 for more information.

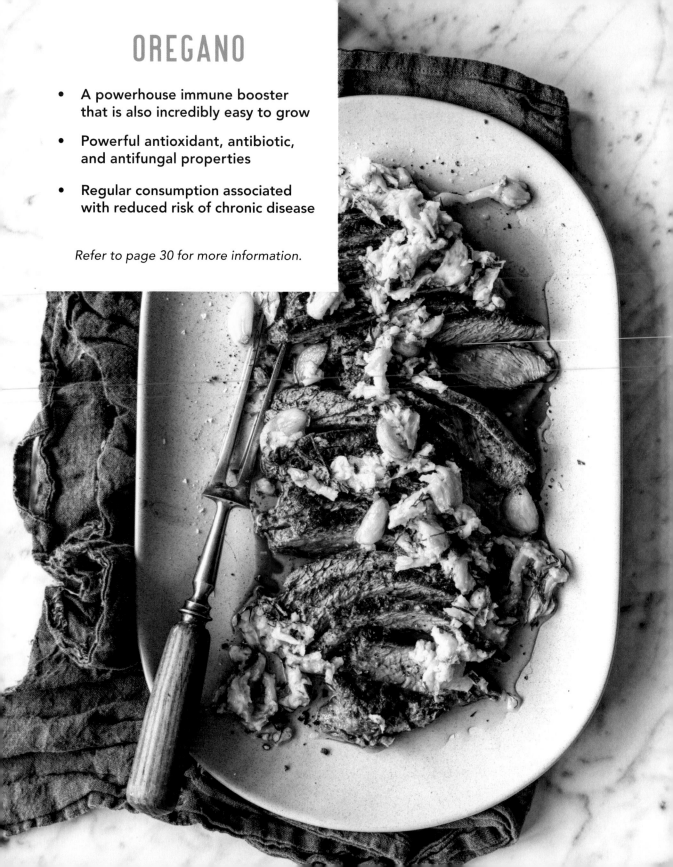

OREGANO

- A powerhouse immune booster that is also incredibly easy to grow

- Powerful antioxidant, antibiotic, and antifungal properties

- Regular consumption associated with reduced risk of chronic disease

Refer to page 30 for more information.

STEAK WITH OREGANO AND ROASTED GARLIC SAUCE

Roasting garlic transforms its bite into velvety sweetness. You might even be tempted to eat this sauce on its own with a spoon! Serve this with your favorite salad (use dandelion greens in the salad to increase this meal's immune-boosting properties even more).

1. Preheat the oven to 350 °F (325 °F convection).

2. To start on the oregano and roasted garlic sauce, peel the outermost papery skin from the garlic bulbs without separating the cloves. Using a sharp knife, cut the tops of the garlic bulbs off, exposing the individual cloves. Place on a baking tray, rub the coconut oil over the cut surfaces of the garlic cloves, then individually wrap each bulb and its chopped-off top in baking paper to create four parcels. Roast for 40 minutes or until the garlic is lightly golden and feels soft when pressed. Set aside to cool a little.

3. When the garlic is cool enough to handle, squeeze the flesh into a bowl and discard the skins. Mash half the garlic with a fork, keeping some cloves chunky. Add the extra-virgin olive oil, lemon juice, oregano, and thyme and mix well. Season with salt and pepper to taste.

4. Use the "hot" setting of an electric griddle, or place a large, heavy frying pan over high heat. Brush the steaks with the remaining coconut oil and season with salt and pepper. Cook the steaks on one side for 1 minute or until brown, then flip and cook for another 1 minute for medium-rare (or cook to your liking). Transfer the steaks to a plate and let them rest for 3 minutes, keeping them warm.

5. Thickly slice the steaks and place them on a platter, spoon the sauce over them, and serve.

Serves: 4

4 thin sirloin steaks (minute steaks), 5 to 6 ounces each

2 tablespoons coconut oil or good-quality animal fat

Sea salt and freshly ground black pepper

OREGANO AND ROASTED GARLIC SAUCE

4 garlic bulbs

1 tablespoon coconut oil

¾ cup extra-virgin olive oil, plus 1 tablespoon for brushing

1 tablespoon lemon juice

Handful oregano leaves, finely chopped

1 teaspoon finely chopped thyme

Sea salt and freshly ground black pepper

NUTRITION INFORMATION: Calories 835.5 | 82.4g total fat (28g saturated fat, 0g trans fat) | 0mg cholesterol | 432.6mg sodium | 9.7g total carbohydrate (0.4g dietary fiber, 5.2g total sugars, 0g added sugars) | 17.9g protein | 0mcg vitamin D | 23.8mg calcium | 1.2mg iron | 305.1mg potassium

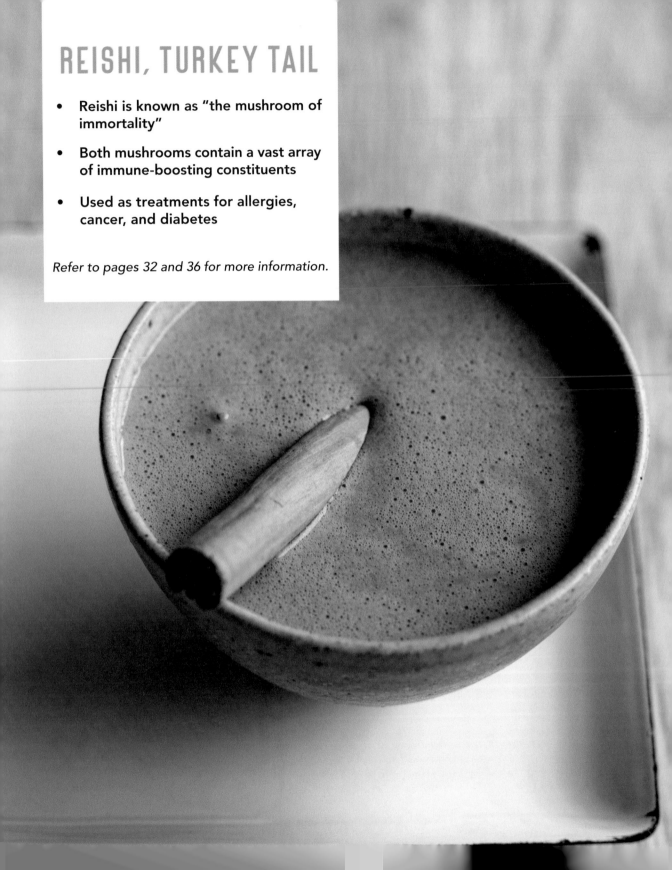

REISHI, TURKEY TAIL

- Reishi is known as "the mushroom of immortality"

- Both mushrooms contain a vast array of immune-boosting constituents

- Used as treatments for allergies, cancer, and diabetes

Refer to pages 32 and 36 for more information.

MUSHROOM LATTE

You may not think that *mushroom* and *latte* should be used in such close proximity to each other, but the sweetness of the cacao, cinnamon, and honey make this a great way to reap the powerful immune-boosting effects of mushrooms—even if you don't typically like their taste.

1. Combine all the ingredients in a small saucepan and stir well.

2. Place over low heat and, while slowly stirring, gently heat until hot.

3. Transfer the hot mixture to a blender. Blend on low, working up to high speed and blending for 1 minute or until foamy.

4. Pour the mixture into a latte glass or a mug and enjoy.

NOTE: If you use coconut milk and find your mushroom latte a little too creamy, stir in some boiling water to reach the consistency you desire. Also, you can use a milk frother instead of a blender to blend your mushroom latte.

Serves: 1

1 cup coconut, hemp, or nut milk

1 teaspoon mushroom powder (reishi, shiitake, turkey tail, lion's mane, chaga, or a blend)

1 teaspoon cacao

¼ teaspoon ground cinnamon

½ to 1 teaspoon manuka honey or other sweetener (optional)

NUTRITION INFORMATION: Calories 65.8 | 5.2g total fat (4.1g saturated fat, 0g trans fat) | 0mg cholesterol | 15.2mg sodium | 4.1g total carbohydrate (2g dietary fiber, 1g total sugars, 0g added sugars) | 0.7g protein | 3mcg vitamin D | 132.6mg calcium | 1.1mg iron | 79mg potassium

RHODIOLA TEA

Because rhodiola is an adaptogen, it's great to drink both when you feel stressed and when you feel lethargic. In either case, it will help bring you back to center while also shoring up your mood and resilience.

Serves: 2

2 tablespoons organic rhodiola tea leaves (see note)

1. Pour 3 cups of boiling water into a teapot or heatproof jar.

2. Stir in the rhodiola tea and let steep for 3 minutes.

3. Strain into mugs and serve.

NOTE: Rhodiola (rose root) can be purchased from health food stores, specialty tea shops, some supermarkets, or online.

NUTRITION INFORMATION: Nutrition information for this recipe is not readily available

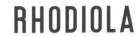

RHODIOLA

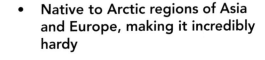

- Native to Arctic regions of Asia and Europe, making it incredibly hardy

- An adaptogen that helps build resilience to physical and mental stress

- Major immune booster with anti-fatigue, antidepressant, antioxidant, anti-inflammatory, anticancer, and antiviral properties

Refer to page 35 for more information.

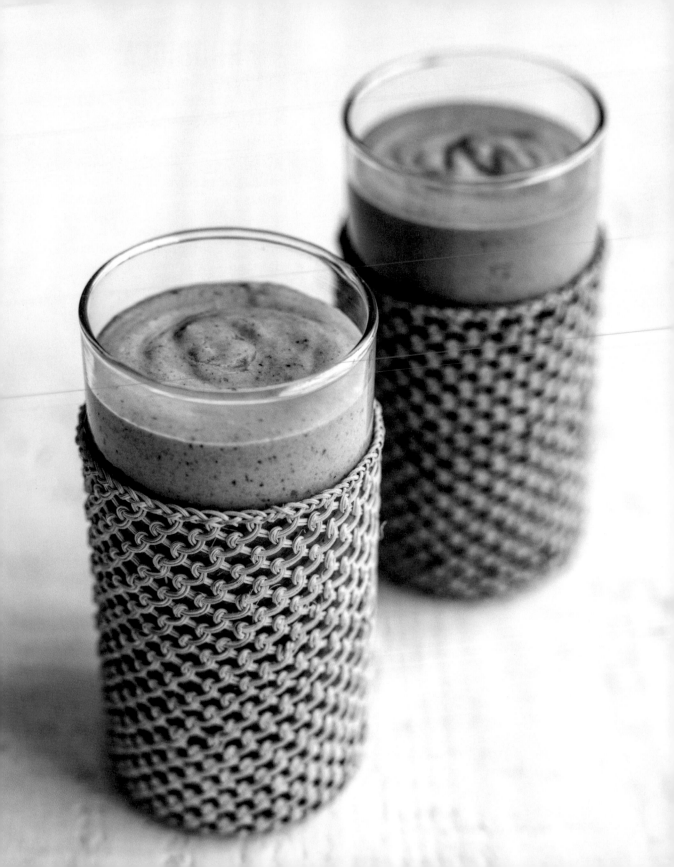

BRAIN-BOOSTING SMOOTHIE

Brain food can be tasty! This delicious smoothie provides healthy fats that fuel your brain, plenty of selenium (from the Brazil nuts), lots of neuroprotective antioxidants in the berries, and rhodiola, which is hailed for its antidepressant properties. If you have any left over, store it in an airtight glass jar in the fridge and have it later in the day for a snack, or the next morning for breakfast—just be sure to consume it within 24 hours.

Place all ingredients in a blender and blend until smooth. Pour into a tall glass (or glasses) and serve.

Serves: 1 to 2

1½ cups hemp milk or other dairy-free milk

1½ cups frozen mixed berries

4 Brazil nuts

½ teaspoon rhodiola powder

1 teaspoon maca power

1 tablespoon collagen powder

1 tablespoon coconut oil or MCT oil

1 tablespoon manuka honey or other sweetener (optional)

NUTRITION INFORMATION: Calories 412.4 | 18.8g total fat (7.6g saturated fat, 0g trans fat) | 0mg cholesterol | 120.2mg sodium | 52.9g total carbohydrate (6.4g dietary fiber, 17.2g total sugars, 16.7g added sugars) | 13.5g protein | 1.9mcg vitamin D | 285.8mg calcium | 1.6mg iron | 119.3mg potassium

MOON DRINK

The moon is gorgeous, mysterious, and illuminating, and so is this drink. Try sipping this concoction in the late afternoons when you need some restoring and you've started to get a little hungry but dinner is still a little ways away. The flavors will keep your tongue guessing, and the heady aroma will coax your mind into a state that allows inspiration to float in.

Serves: 2

2½ cups unsweetened dairy-free milk (such as hemp, macadamia, or coconut milk)

¼ teaspoon ground cinnamon

¼ teaspoon ground turmeric

2 pinches ground cardamom

¼ teaspoon ground ginger

½ teaspoon ground ashwagandha

½ teaspoon extra-virgin coconut oil (optional)

Manuka honey or other sweetener

Freshly cracked black pepper

Cinnamon stick, finely grated, or a pinch of ground cinnamon (optional)

1. Place the dairy-free milk in a small saucepan over medium-low heat.

2. Add the spices and ashwagandha and heat, gently stirring, for 5 minutes or until it is heated through and the flavor has developed.

3. Stir in the coconut oil, if using, and honey to taste.

4. Pour into mugs and sprinkle with some freshly cracked black pepper.

5. Top with finely grated cinnamon, if using, then slowly sip and enjoy.

NUTRITION INFORMATION: Calories 142.6 | 8.1g total fat (7.2g saturated fat, 0g trans fat) | 0mg cholesterol | 20mg sodium | 19.9g total carbohydrate (6.9g dietary fiber, 9.5g total sugars, 0g added sugars) | 1.2g protein | 3.8mcg vitamin D | 247.5mg calcium | 2.2mg iron | 147.5mg potassium

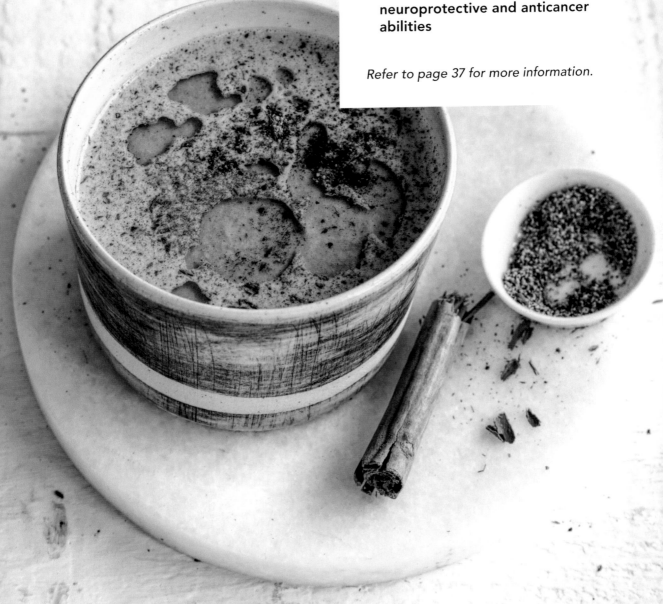

TURMERIC

- Major anti-inflammatory with a broad positive effect on immune function

- Found to be helpful in numerous conditions and diseases—too many to list

- Recent research focuses on neuroprotective and anticancer abilities

Refer to page 37 for more information.

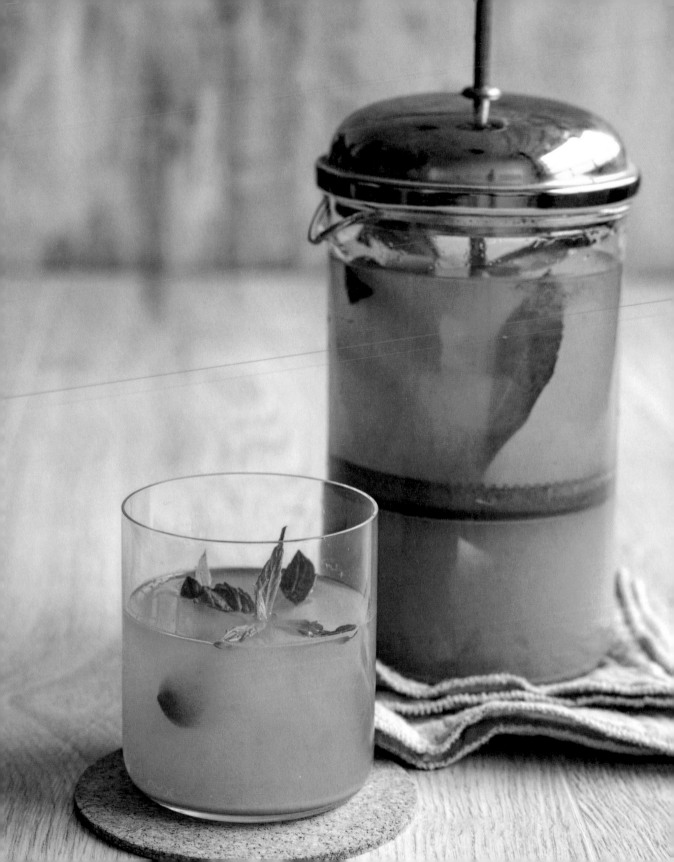

TURMERIC AND COCONUT TONIC

Sometimes we all need a pick-me-up. This tonic delivers a ton more health benefits than a tall glass of lemonade—and just as much taste. The cayenne pepper will really get you going, but it can be irritating to the gut, so definitely skip it if you're paying extra attention to healing your digestive tract.

1. Place the coconut water, ginger, lemon juice, turmeric, manuka honey, and cayenne pepper (if using) in a large (8-cup) plunger jar with the plunger strainer completely removed, or use a large mason jar with a lid.

2. Stir well, cover, and refrigerate overnight.

3. The next day, insert the plunger strainer into the jar and gently press down so the pulp remains on the bottom, or strain the liquid through a fine sieve and discard the ginger pulp.

4. Mix in a handful of mint leaves and serve chilled with ice.

Serves: 4

4 cups coconut water

1 tablespoon finely grated ginger

Juice of 1 lemon

1 tablespoon finely grated fresh turmeric

1 to 2 tablespoons manuka honey

1 to 2 pinches cayenne pepper (optional)

1 handful fresh mint leaves

NUTRITION INFORMATION: Calories 99.2 | 0.7g total fat (0.5g saturated fat, 0g trans fat) | 0mg cholesterol | 68.7mg sodium | 21.7g total carbohydrate (3.7g dietary fiber, 15.7g total sugars, 0g added sugars) | 2.3g protein | 0mcg vitamin D | 24.6mg calcium | 1.7mg iron | 514.5mg potassium

TURMERIC ELIXIR

Are you ready to spice up your medicine cabinet? This feisty elixir delivers a major dose of anti-inflammatory power thanks to turmeric and ginger. The freshly ground black pepper increases the bioavailability of the curcumin in the turmeric, so don't skip that part. Besides, the black pepper gives this mixture that much more of a kick! (Don't worry, the honey and cinnamon balance everything out in a lovely way.) Take 1½ tablespoons up to three times a day.

Makes: 2 cups

1 pound fresh turmeric

10 ounces ginger

2½ tablespoons filtered water

2 teaspoons manuka honey or monk fruit sweetener, or to taste

¼ teaspoon ground cinnamon

Pinch freshly ground black pepper

1. You'll need a mason jar with a lid for this recipe. Wash the jar in very hot water or run it through a hot rinse cycle in the dishwasher.

2. Juice the turmeric and ginger in a cold-press juicer.

3. Mix in the water, honey, cinnamon, and pepper and pour into the sterilized jar. Cover and allow to steep for 1 hour before using.

4. Store the turmeric elixir in the fridge for up to 5 days.

NUTRITION INFORMATION: Calories 130.1 | 1.4g total fat (0.8g saturated fat, 0g trans fat) | 0mg cholesterol | 10.8mg sodium | 28g total carbohydrate (7.8g dietary fiber, 1.7g total sugars, 0g added sugars) | 3.8g protein | 0mcg vitamin D | 59.4mg calcium | 16.7mg iron | 718.2mg potassium

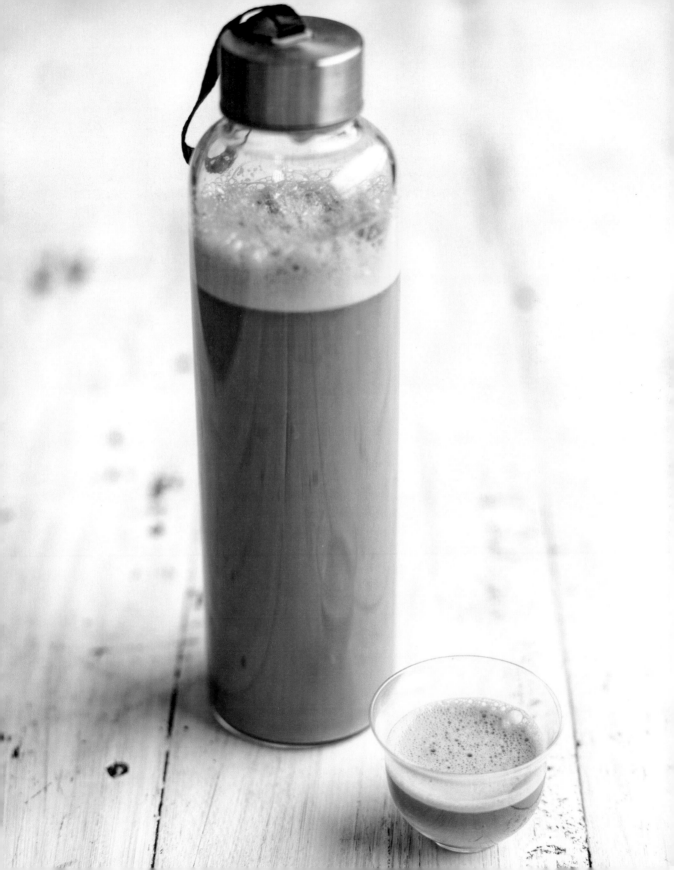

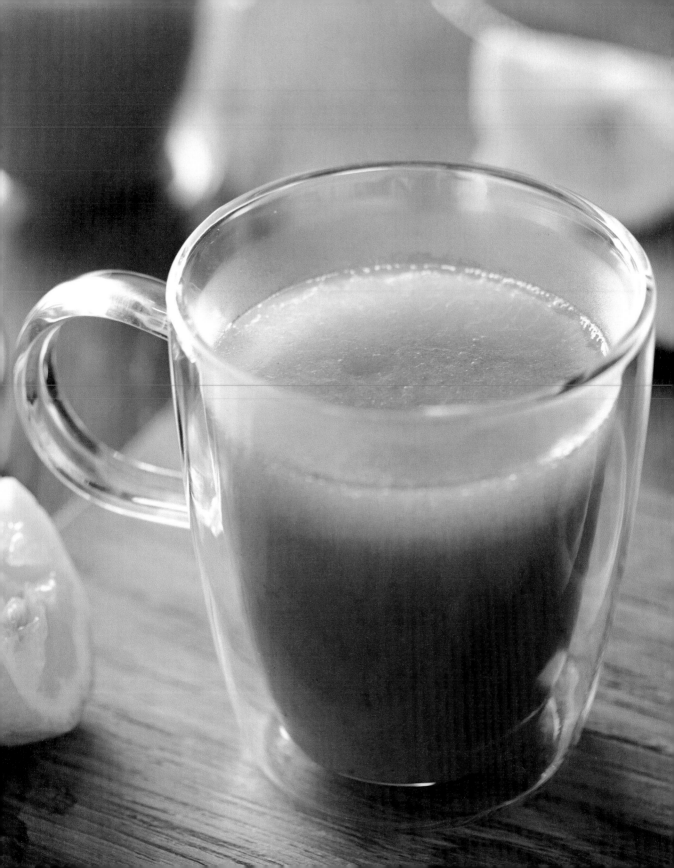

BONE BROTH
WITH TURMERIC, LEMON, AND CUMIN

I have a vision for the future, and it involves everyone drinking bone broths daily instead of coffee! After all, we need to do something to address our modern-day health problems, and one of the best ways to start is by healing the gut. Bone broths do just that and are also pretty delicious. This recipe is infused with turmeric as well as some lemon juice. Drink a cup a day!

1. Pour the hot broth into a large mug.

2. Add the turmeric, cumin, lemon juice, and a pinch of salt and give it a good stir.

3. Take a sip and enjoy at any time of day.

Serves: 1

1½ cups hot fish broth, beef broth, or Chicken Bone Broth (page 146)

1 teaspoon ground turmeric

Pinch ground cumin

2 teaspoons lemon juice, or to taste

Sea salt

NUTRITION INFORMATION: Calories 49.1 | 0.6g total fat (0.1g saturated fat, 0g trans fat) | 0mg cholesterol | 698mg sodium | 4.4g total carbohydrate (0.9g dietary fiber, 1.1g total sugars, 0.7g added sugars) | 7.6g protein | 0mcg vitamin D | 45.8mg calcium | 4.2mg iron | 754.9mg potassium

CHICKEN BONE BROTH

All around the world, chicken broth is hailed for its immune-boosting properties. It's also delicious and extremely nourishing to the gut. You'll want to have some of this healing liquid always on hand, both to drink on its own and to use as a base for healthful and flavorful soups. After you've made it just a few times, this recipe will become second nature and you won't even have to refer to this book.

Makes: 3½ to 4 quarts

2½ pounds bony chicken parts (such as necks, backs, breast bones, and wings)

2 to 4 chicken feet (optional)

2 tablespoons apple cider vinegar

1 large onion, roughly chopped

2 carrots, roughly chopped

3 celery stalks, roughly chopped

2 leeks (white part only), roughly chopped

1 garlic bulb, cut in half horizontally

1 tablespoon black peppercorns, lightly crushed

2 bay leaves

2 large handfuls flat-leaf parsley stalks

Filtered water

1. Place the chicken parts in a stockpot. Add all the ingredients and 5 quarts of cold filtered water and let stand for 1½ hours to help draw out the nutrients from the bones.

2. Place the pot over medium-high heat and bring to a boil, skimming off any scum that forms on the surface of the liquid. Reduce the heat to low and simmer for 12 to 24 hours. The longer you cook the broth, the richer and more flavorful it will be.

3. Strain the broth through a fine sieve into a large container, cover, and place in the fridge overnight so the fat rises to the top and congeals. Skim off the fat and reserve for cooking; it will keep in the fridge for up to 1 week or in the freezer for up to 3 months.

4. Transfer the broth to smaller airtight containers. The broth can be stored in the fridge for 3 to 4 days or in the freezer for up to 3 months.

NUTRITION INFORMATION: Calories 52.3 | 2.9g total fat (0.9g saturated fat, 0g trans fat) | 2.6mg cholesterol | 341.5mg sodium | 0.9g total carbohydrate (0g dietary fiber, 0.4g total sugars, 0g added sugars) | 5.3g protein | 0.1mcg vitamin D | 10.6mg calcium | 0.5mg iron | 205.7mg potassium

MISCELLANEOUS

- The recipes in the pages ahead don't use any one particular herb. Rather, they include drinks to support a healthy lifestyle and build immunity, along with delicious foods that will likely become staples of your menu.

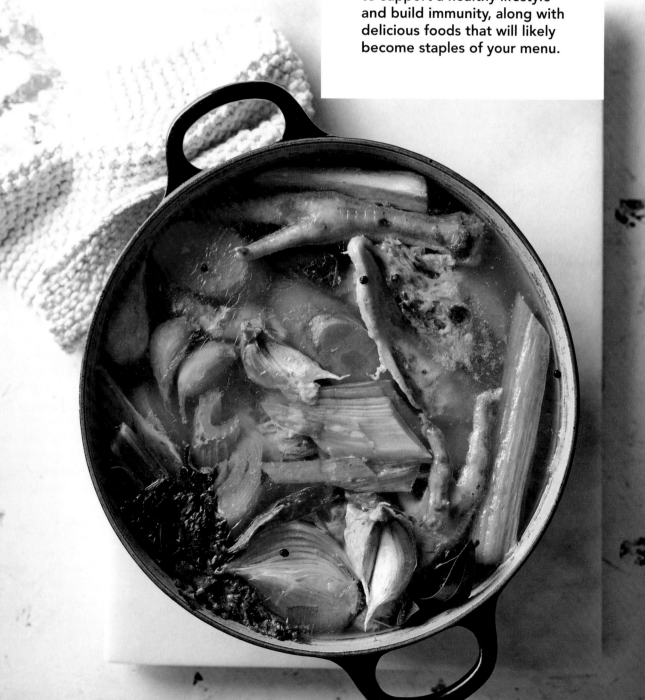

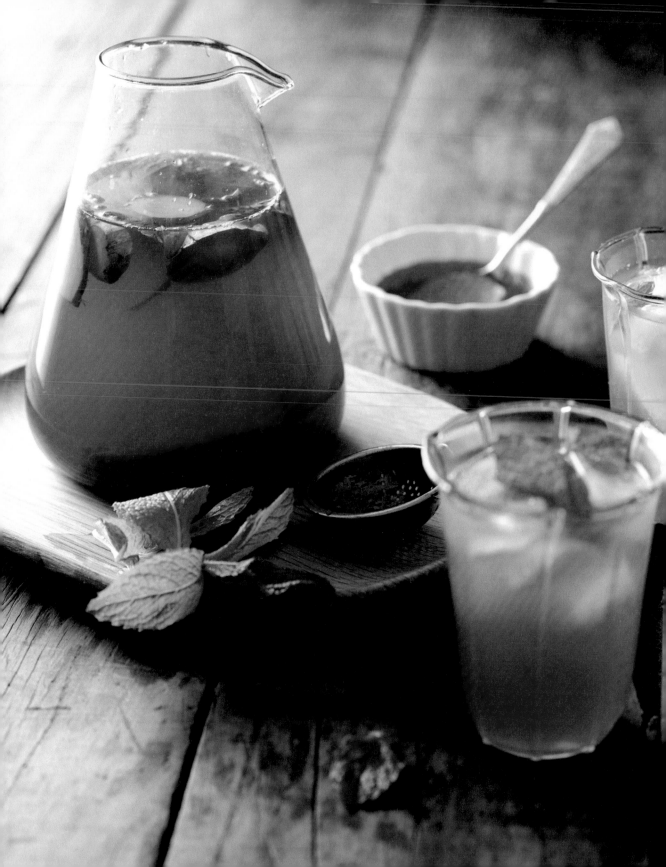

SALT WATER FLUSH

There are times when you might experience constipation, or just a sense of wanting to clean out your digestive system. This salt water flush will help you do just that. Since 80 percent of your immune system is in your gut, this digestive reset will also help unburden many of your mechanisms of immunity and increase your resilience. Definitely don't drink this on your way out the door—you should feel a strong urge to use the bathroom within 30 minutes of downing it.

Stir the warm water, salt, and lemon juice together and drink quickly on an empty stomach within 30 minutes of waking. Food or other drinks should not be consumed until at least 30 to 60 minutes later.

Serves: 1

4 cups warm filtered water

2 teaspoons Himalayan salt or sea salt

2 to 3 tablespoons lemon juice, or to taste

NUTRITION INFORMATION: Calories 0.7 | 0g total fat (0g saturated fat, 0g trans fat) | 0mg cholesterol | 4416mg sodium | 0.2g total carbohydrate (0g dietary fiber, 0.1g total sugars, 0g added sugars) | 0g protein | 0mcg vitamin D | 19.4mg calcium | 0.4mg iron | 36.7mg potassium

LEMON WATER

This recipe relies on the single most important ingredient in this whole book: clean, filtered water! I drink at least 2 liters of water a day, and I always start with at least 16 ounces during the first 10 to 20 minutes after I wake up, as that is when our bodies are most dehydrated. Room-temperature water is ideal because it doesn't shock your system too much. Lemon juice has antifungal and antibacterial properties; it's also anti-inflammatory and a good source of vitamin C and potassium. Apple cider vinegar has a beneficial effect on blood sugar levels, boosts detoxification, and promotes circulation of your lymphatic system, which is an important component of the immune system.

Serves: 1

4 cups room-temperature or luke-warm filtered water

Juice of 1 lemon or 2 tablespoons apple cider vinegar

1. Stir the water and lemon juice together and drink, on an empty stomach, within 30 minutes of waking.

2. Food or other drinks should not be consumed until at least 30 to 60 minutes later.

NUTRITION INFORMATION: Calories 24.4 | 0.3g total fat (0g saturated fat, 0g trans fat) | 0mg cholesterol | 1.7mg sodium | 7.8g total carbohydrate (2.4g dietary fiber, 2.1g total sugars, 0g added sugars) | 0.9g protein | 0mcg vitamin D | 21.8mg calcium | 0.5mg iron | 115.9mg potassium

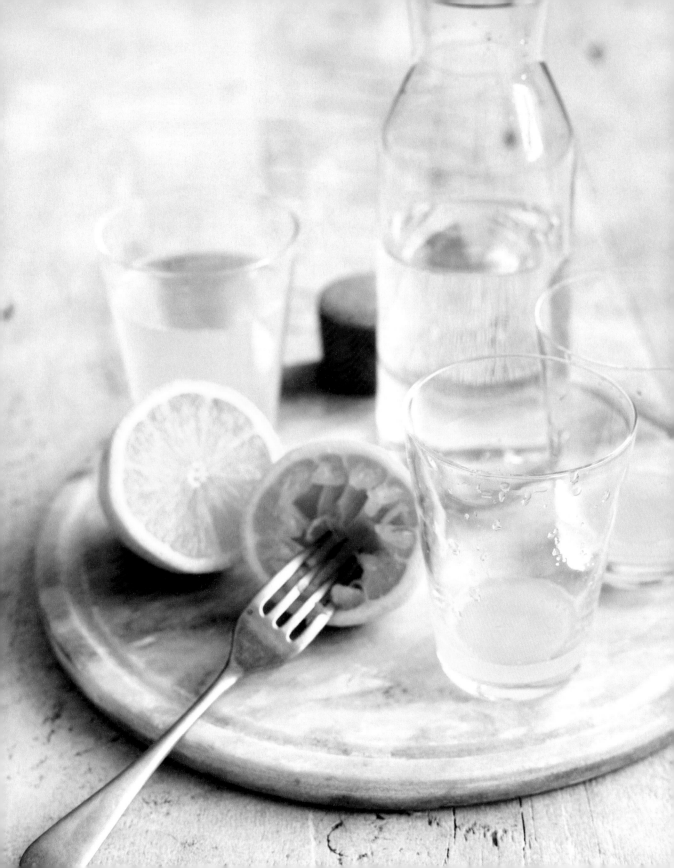

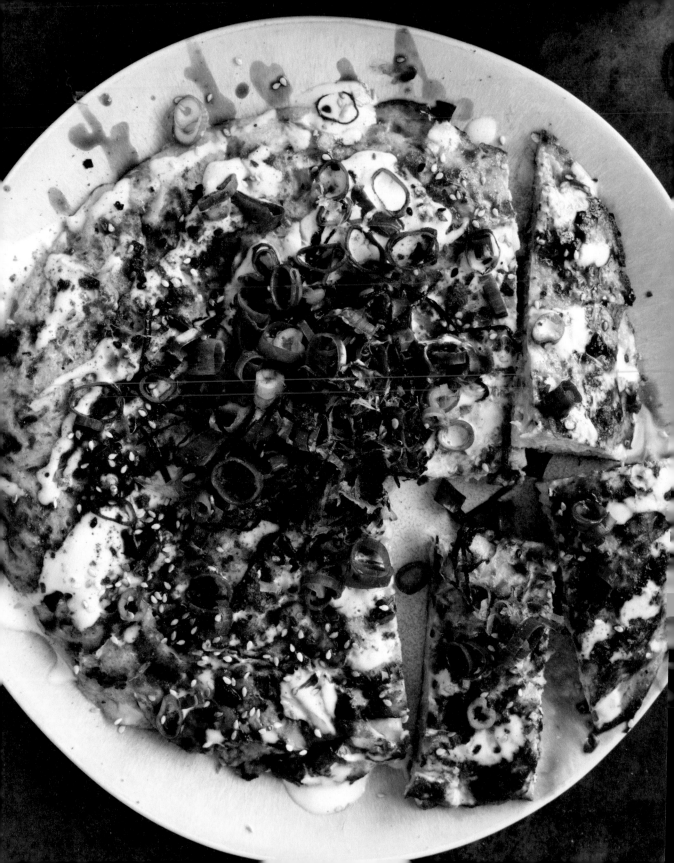

JAPANESE PANCAKES

Okay, these aren't particularly immune boosting (although the green cabbage is a cruciferous vegetable, nutrient rich). They're just so tasty, I had to include a recipe for them.

Also known as okonomiyaki, these ever-delightful Japanese cabbage pancakes will have the most hardened cabbage hater lining up for more. These pancakes are so more-ish (meaning, they make you want more), they defy logic. The charred cabbage, mayonnaise, and seaweed make for a perfect flavor combination. You can add seafood or bacon if you feel like a bit of meat, or simply add some mushrooms or carrots to stay on the vegetarian train. My advice is to make a heap of these, as leftovers are a perfect lunch the next day.

1. Whisk the eggs, coconut flour, baking powder, tamari, and sesame oil in a bowl until there are no lumps.

2. Add the cabbage and the white part of the spring onions and mix well to combine. Season with a little salt and pepper.

3. Heat a large nonstick frying pan over medium heat and add 1 tablespoon of oil. Ladle in a quarter of the batter—about ½ cup—and spread out gently with the back of a spoon until about 5 inches in diameter. Cook the pancake for 2 minutes or until the top dries slightly and the bottom starts to brown.

4. Flip and cook for an additional 2 minutes. Transfer to a serving plate.

5. Repeat with the remaining oil and pancake batter to make four pancakes.

6. Top each pancake with a drizzle of teriyaki sauce and a dollop of mayonnaise, then sprinkle on the green part of the spring onion, nori, shichimi togarashi, and bonito flakes.

Serves: 4

6 eggs

2 tablespoons coconut flour

1 teaspoon baking powder

1 tablespoon tamari or coconut aminos

½ teaspoon toasted sesame oil

¾ cup green cabbage, finely shredded on a mandoline

2 spring onions, white and green parts separated, thinly sliced

Sea salt and freshly ground black pepper

⅓ cup melted coconut oil or good-quality animal fat

TO SERVE

½ cup Teriyaki Sauce (page 154)

¾ cup Japanese Mayonnaise (page 154)

1 sheet toasted nori, thinly sliced

1 to 1½ teaspoons shichimi togarashi (Japanese 7-spice blend), or to taste

2 tablespoons bonito flakes

NUTRITION INFORMATION: Calories 513.4 | 44.3g total fat (20.9g saturated fat, 0g trans fat) | 246.3mg cholesterol | 1768.9mg sodium | 16.8g total carbohydrate (3.7g dietary fiber, 7.1g total sugars, 3.1g added sugars) | 12.2g protein | 1.4mcg vitamin D | 128.4mg calcium | 1.8mg iron | 256.6mg potassium

JAPANESE MAYONNAISE

Makes: 2 cups

4 egg yolks

2 teaspoons Dijon mustard

1½ tablespoons apple cider vinegar

1 teaspoon tamari or coconut aminos

¼ teaspoon garlic powder

Sea salt and freshly ground black pepper

1½ cups olive or macadamia oil (or ¾ cup of each)

1. Place the egg yolks, mustard, vinegar, tamari, garlic powder, and a pinch of salt in a glass jar and blend with a handheld blender until smooth and creamy. (Alternatively, place in the bowl of a food processor and process until combined.)

2. With the processor running, slowly pour in the oil in a thin, steady stream and process until the mayonnaise is thick and creamy.

3. Season with additional salt and pepper to taste. Store in a sealed glass jar in the fridge for up to 5 days.

NUTRITION INFORMATION (for full recipe): Calories 824.3 | 91.3g total fat (14g saturated fat, 0g trans fat) | 170mg cholesterol | 177.8mg sodium | 1g total carbohydrate (0.1g dietary fiber, 0.2g total sugars, 0g added sugars) | 2.8g protein | 0mcg vitamin D | 22.6mg calcium | 0.5mg iron | 31.2mg potassium

TERIYAKI SAUCE

Makes: ⁴/₅ cup

½ cup tamari or coconut aminos

3 tablespoons coconut sugar

3 tablespoons honey

2 teaspoons finely grated garlic

1 teaspoon finely grated ginger

1½ teaspoons tapioca flour

1. Mix the tamari, sugar, honey, garlic, ginger, and 3 tablespoons of water in a small saucepan and place over medium heat. Bring to a boil, then reduce the heat to low and gently simmer for 5 minutes to dissolve the sugar and allow the flavors to develop.

2. Meanwhile, mix the tapioca flour and 1 tablespoon of water until smooth.

3. Bring the tamari mixture to a boil, then pour in the tapioca mixture. Stir constantly until the sauce is thickened and coats the back of the spoon. Remove from the heat.

4. Allow to cool, then strain, discarding the ginger and garlic pulp.

5. Store in an airtight glass jar in the fridge for up to 4 weeks.

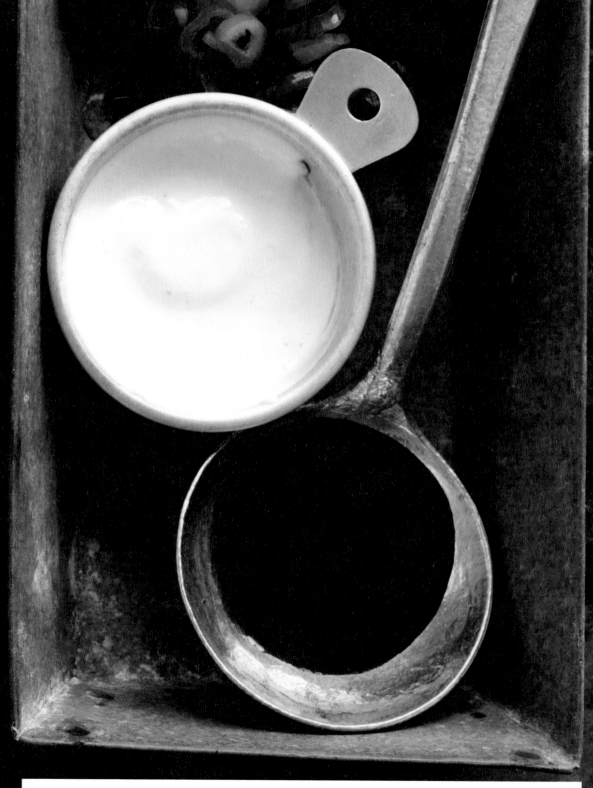

NUTRITION INFORMATION: Calories 110.9 | 0.1g total fat (0g saturated fat, 0g trans fat) | 0mg cholesterol | 2027.6mg sodium | 25.5g total carbohydrate (0.4g dietary fiber, 22.7g total sugars, 22g added sugars) | 3.9g protein | 0mcg vitamin D | 8.8mg calcium | 1mg iron | 140mg potassium

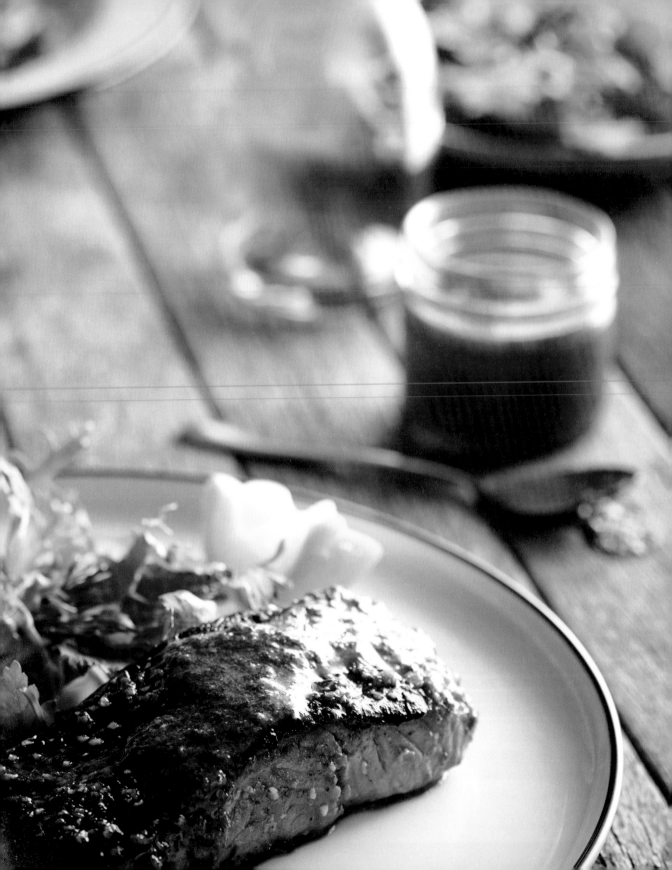

HERB AND ANCHOVY DRESSING

Put the parsley, dill, chives, anchovies, and vinegar in a food processor bowl or high-speed blender jug and process until combined. With the motor running, slowly pour in the oil and process until smooth. Pour the dressing into a bowl and season with salt and pepper. Store in the fridge for up to 3 days.

2 large handfuls of flat-leaf parsley leaves, roughly chopped

1 handful of dill fronds, roughly chopped

3 tablespoons snipped chives

2 salted anchovy fillets, rinsed and patted dry

2 tablespoons apple cider vinegar

1½ cups extra-virgin olive oil

Sea salt and freshly ground black pepper

NUTRITION INFORMATION: Calories 247.6 | 27.9g total fat (8.7g saturated fat, 0g trans fat) | .4mg cholesterol | 50.1mg sodium | 2.8g total carbohydrate (.5g dietary fiber, 0.1g total sugars, 0g added sugars) | .5g protein | 0mcg vitamin D | 33.1mg calcium | 1.4mg iron | 123.9mg potassium)

METRIC CONVERSION CHART

The recipes in this book use the standard United States method for measuring liquid and dry or solid ingredients (teaspoons, tablespoons, and cups). The following charts are provided to help cooks outside the U.S. successfully use these recipes. All equivalents are approximate.

Standard Cup	Fine Powder (e.g., flour)	Grain (e.g., rice)	Granular (e.g., sugar)	Liquid Solids (e.g., butter)	Liquid (e.g., milk)
1	140 g	150 g	190 g	200 g	240 ml
¾	105 g	113 g	143 g	150 g	180 ml
⅔	93 g	100 g	125 g	133 g	160 ml
½	70 g	75 g	95 g	100 g	120 ml
⅓	47 g	50 g	63 g	67 g	80 ml
¼	35 g	38 g	48 g	50 g	60 ml
⅛	18 g	19 g	24 g	25 g	30 ml

Useful Equivalents for Liquid Ingredients by Volume			
¼ tsp			1 ml
½ tsp			2 ml
1 tsp			5 ml
3 tsp	1 tbsp	½ fl oz	15 ml
	2 tbsp	⅛ cup	1 fl oz	30 ml
	4 tbsp	¼ cup	2 fl oz	60 ml
	5⅓ tbsp	⅓ cup	3 fl oz	80 ml
	8 tbsp	½ cup	4 fl oz	120 ml
	10⅔ tbsp	⅔ cup	5 fl oz	160 ml
	12 tbsp	¾ cup	6 fl oz	180 ml
	16 tbsp	1 cup	8 fl oz	240 ml
	1 pt	2 cups	16 fl oz	480 ml
	1 qt	4 cups	32 fl oz	960 ml
			33 fl oz	1000 ml	1 L

Useful Equivalents for Dry Ingredients by Weight		
(To convert ounces to grams, multiply the number of ounces by 30.)		
1 oz	¹⁄₁₆ lb	30 g
4 oz	¼ lb	120 g
8 oz	½ lb	240 g
12 oz	¾ lb	360 g
16 oz	1 lb	480 g

Useful Equivalents for Cooking/Oven Temperatures			
Process	Fahrenheit	Celsius	Gas Mark
Freeze Water	32 °F	0 °C	
Room Temperature	68 °F	20 °C	
Boil Water	212 °F	100 °C	
Bake	325 °F	160 °C	3
	350 °F	180 °C	4
	375 °F	190 °C	5
	400 °F	200 °C	6
	425 °F	220 °C	7
	450 °F	230 °C	8
Broil			Grill

Useful Equivalents for Length				
(To convert inches to centimeters, multiply the number of inches by 2.5.)				
1 in			2.5 cm	
6 in	½ ft		15 cm	
12 in	1 ft		30 cm	
36 in	3 ft	1 yd	90 cm	
40 in			100 cm	1 m

ENDNOTES

The Benefits of Herbs and Spices

1. M. Darooghegi Mofrad et al., "Garlic Supplementation Reduces Circulating C-reactive Protein, Tumor Necrosis Factor, and Interleukin-6 in Adults: A Systematic Review and Meta-analysis of Randomized Controlled Trials," *Journal of Nutrition* 149, no. 4 (2019): 605–618. https://doi.org/10.1093/jn/nxy310.

2. V. Vaidya, K. Ingold, and D. Pratt, "Garlic: Source of the Ultimate Antioxidants—Sulfenic Acids," *Angewadte Chemie International Edition* 48, no. 1 (2008): 157–60. https://doi.org/10.1002/anie.200804560.

3. B. Mafuvadze et al., "Apigenin Induces Apoptosis and Blocks Growth of Medroxyprogesterone Acetate-Dependent BT-474 Xenograft Tumors," *Hormones & Cancer* 3, no. 4 (2012): 160–71. https://doi.org/10.1007/s12672-012-0114-x.

4. E. Riza et al., "The Effect of Greek Herbal Tea Consumption on Thyroid Cancer: A Case-Control Study," *European Journal of Public Health* 25, no. 6 (2015): 1001–05. https://doi.org/10.1093/eurpub/ckv063.

5. B. B. Aggarwal et al., "Identification of Novel Anti-Inflammatory Agents from Ayurvedic Medicine for Prevention of Chronic Diseases: 'Reverse Pharmacology' and 'Bedside to Bench' Approach," *Current Drug Targets* 12, no. 1 (2011): 1595–1653. https://doi.org/10.2174/138945011798109464.

6. F. Yang et al., "Curcumin Inhibits Formation of Amyloid Beta Oligomers and Fibrils, Binds Plaques, and Reduces Amyloid In Vivo," *Journal of Biological Chemistry* 280, no. 7 (2005): 5892–901. https://doi.org/10.1074/jbc.M404751200.

7. A. N. Hoehn and A. L. Stockert, "The Effects of Cinnamomum Cassia on Blood Glucose Values Are Greater than Those of Dietary Changes Alone," *Nutrition and Metabolic Insights* 5 (2012): 77–83. https://doi.org/10.4137/NMI.S10498.

8. T. Perrinjaquet-Moccetti et al., "Food Supplementation with an Olive (*Olea Europaea L.*) Leaf Extract Reduces Blood Pressure in Borderline Hypertensive Monozygotic Twins," *Phytotherapy Research: PTR* 22, no. 9 (2008): 1239–42. https://doi.org/10.1002/ptr.2455.

9. J. Hancke et al., "A Double-Blind Study with a New Monodrug Kan Jang: Decrease of Symptoms and Improvement in the Recovery from Common Colds," *Phytotherapy Research* 9, no. 8 (1995): 559–62. https://doi.org/10.1002/ptr.2650090804.

10. D. D. Cáceres et al., "Prevention of Common Colds with Andrographis Paniculata Dried Extract. A Pilot Double Blind Trial," *Phytomedicine* 4, no. 2 (1997): 101–4. https://doi.org/10.1016/S0944-7113(97)80051-7.

11. H. C. Ko, B. L. Wei, and W. F. Chiou, "The Effect of Medicinal Plants Used in Chinese Folk Medicine on RANTES Secretion by Virus-Infected Human Epithelial Cells," *Journal of Ethnopharmacology* 107, no. 2 (2006): 205–10. https://doi.org/10.1016/j.jep.2006.03.004.

12. L. L. Kulichenko et al., "A Randomized, Controlled Study of Kan Jang Versus Amantadine in the Treatment of Influenza in Volgograd," *Journal of Herbal Pharmacotherapy* 3, no. 1 (2003): 77–93. https://pubmed.ncbi.nlm.nih.gov/15277072.

13. A. Puri et al., "Immunostimulant Agents from *Andrographis paniculate*," *Journal of Natural Products* 56, no. 7 (1993): 995–99. https://doi/org/10.1021/np50097a002.

14. J. Salve et al., "Adaptogenic and Anxiolytic Effects of Ashwagandha Root Extract in Healthy Adults: A Double-Blind, Randomized, Placebo-Controlled Clinical Study," *Cureus* 11, no. 12 (2019): e6466. https://doi.org/10.7759/cureus.6466.

15. W. C. Huang et al., "Astragalus Polysaccharide (PG2) Ameliorates Cancer Symptom Clusters, as Well as Improves Quality of Life in Patients with Metastatic Disease, Through Modulation of the Inflammatory Cascade," *Cancers* 11, no 8 (2019): 1054. https://doi.org/10.3390/cancers11081054.

16. G. Su et al., "Oral Astragalus (Huang Qi) for Preventing Frequent Episodes of Acute Respiratory Tract Infection in Children," *Cochrane Database of Systematic Reviews* 12, no. 12 (2016): CD011958. https://doi.org/10.1002/14651858.CD011958.pub2; Z. Guo et al., "A Systematic Review of Phytochemistry, Pharmacology and Pharmacokinetics on *Astragali* Radix: Implications for *Astragali* Radix as a Personalized Medicine," *International Journal of Molecular Sciences* 20, no. 6 (2019): 1463. https://doi.org/10.3390/ijms20061463.

17. S. Alsuhaibani and M. A. Khan, "Immune-Stimulatory and Therapeutic Activity of *Tinospora cordifolia*: Double-Edged Sword against Salmonellosis," *Journal of Immunology Research*. 2017, article 1787803. https://doi.org/10.1155/2017/1787803.

18. A. Gupta et al., "Evaluation of *Cyavanaprāśa* on Health and Immunity Related Parameters in Healthy Children: A Two Arm, Randomized, Open Labeled, Prospective, Multicenter, Clinical Study," *Ancient Science of Life* 36, no. 3 (2017): 141–50. https://doi.org/10.4103/asl.ASL_8_17.

19. J. Sastry et al., "Quantification of Immunity Status of Dabur Chyawanprash: A Review Part-1 (Experimental Studies)," *Indian Journal of Applied Research* 4, no. 2 (2014): 20–24. https://doi.org/10.15373/2249555X/FEB2014/131.

20. K. Díaz et al., "Isolation and Identification of Compounds from Bioactive Extracts of *Taraxacum officinale* Weber ex F. H. Wigg. (Dandelion) as a Potential Source of Antibacterial Agents," *Evidence-Based Complementary and Alternative Medicine: eCAM*, 2018, article 2706417. https://doi.org/10.1155/2018/2706417.

21. H. Han et al., "Inhibitory Effect of Aqueous Dandelion Extract on HIV-1 Replication and Reverse Transcriptase Activity," *BMC Complementary and Alternative Medicine* 11 (2011): 112. https://doi.org/10.1186/1472-6882-11-112.

22. Y. Y. Jia et al., "Taraxacum mongolicum Extract Exhibits a Protective Effect on Hepatocytes and an Antiviral Effect against Hepatitis B Virus in Animal and Human Cells," *Molecular Medicine Reports* 9, no. 4 (2014): 1381–87. https://doi.org/10.3892/mmr.2014.1925.

23. S. C. Sigstedt et al., "Evaluation of Aqueous Extracts of Taraxacum Officinale on Growth and Invasion of Breast and Prostate Cancer Cells," *International Journal of Oncology* 32, no. 5 (2008): 1085–90. https://pubmed.ncbi.nlm.nih.gov/18425335.

24. M. González-Castejón, F. Visioli, and A. Rodriguez-Casado, "Diverse Biological Activities of Dandelion," *Nutrition Reviews* 70, no. 9 (2012): 534–47. https://doi.org/10.1111/j.1753-4887.2012.00509.x.

25. K. I. Block and M. N. Mead, "Immune System Effects of Echinacea, Ginseng, and Astragalus: A Review," *Integrative Cancer Therapies* 2, no. 3 (2003): 247–67. https://doi.org/10.1177/1534735403256419.

26. M. Catanzaro et al., "Immunomodulators Inspired by Nature: A Review on Curcumin and Echinacea," *Molecules* 23, no. 11 (2018): 2778. https://doi.org/10.3390/molecules23112778.

27. K. I. Block and M. N. Mead, " Immune System Effects of Echinacea, Ginseng, and Astragalus: A Review," *Integrative Cancer Therapies* 2, no. 3 (2003): 247–67. https://doi.org/10.1177/1534735403256419.

28. K. Rauš et al., "Effect of an Echinacea-Based Hot Drink Versus Oseltamivir in Influenza Treatment: A Randomized, Double-Blind, Double-Dummy, Multicenter, Noninferiority Clinical Trial," *Current Therapeutic Research, Clinical and Experimental* 77 (2015): 66–72. https://doi.org/10.1016/j.curtheres.2015.04.001.

29. S. Pleschka et al., "Anti-Viral Properties and Mode of Action of Standardized *Echinacea purpurea* Extract Against Highly Pathogenic Avian Influenza Virus (H5N1, H7N7) and Swine-Origin H1N1 (S-OIV)," *Virology Journal* 6 (2009): 197. https://doi.org/10.1186/1743-422X-6-197.

30. V. Barak, T. Halperin, and I. Kalickman, "The Effect of Sambucol, a Black Elderberry-Based, Natural Product, on the Production of Human Cytokines: I. Inflammatory Cytokines," *European Cytokine Network* 12, no. 2 (2001): 290–96.

31. Z. Zakay-Rones et al., "Randomized Study of the Efficacy and Safety of Oral Elderberry Extract in the Treatment of Influenza A and B Virus Infections," *Journal of International Medical Research* 32, no. 2 (2004): 132–40. https://doi.org/10.1177/147323000403200205.

32. R. S. Porter and R. F. Bode, "A Review of the Antiviral Properties of Black Elder (*Sambucus nigra L.*) Products," *Phytotherapy Research* 31, no. 4 (2017): 533–54. https://doi.org/10.1002/ptr.5782.

33. E. Tiralongo, S. S. Wee, and R. A. Lea, "Elderberry Supplementation Reduces Cold Duration and Symptoms in Air-Travellers: A Randomized, Double-Blind Placebo-Controlled Clinical Trial," *Nutrients* 8, no. 4 (2016): 182. https://doi.org/10.3390/nu8040182.

34. G. Goncagul and E. Ayaz, "Antimicrobial Effect of Garlic (Allium sativum)," *Recent Patents on Anti-Infective Drug Discovery* 5, no. 1 (2010): 91–93. https://doi.org/10.2174/157489110790112536.

35. M. P. Nantz et al., "Supplementation with Aged Garlic Extract Improves Both NK and γδ-T Cell Function and Reduces the Severity of Cold and Flu Symptoms: A Randomized, Double-Blind, Placebo-Controlled Nutrition Intervention," *Clinical Nutrition* 31, no. 3 (2012): 337–44. https://doi.org/10.1016/j.clnu.2011.11.019.

36. G. Goncagul and E. Ayaz, "Antimicrobial Effect of Garlic (Allium sativum)," *Recent Patents on Anti-Infective Drug Discovery* 5, no. 1 (2010): 91–93. https://doi.org/10.2174/157489110790112536.

37. M. T. Sultan et al., "Immunity: Plants as Effective Mediators," *Critical Reviews in Food Science and Nutrition* 54, no. 10 (2014): 1298–308. https://doi.org/10.1080/10408398.2011.633249.

38. N. Aryaeian et al., "The Effect of Ginger Supplementation on Some Immunity and Inflammation Intermediate Genes Expression in Patients with Active Rheumatoid Arthritis," *Gene* 698 (2019): 179–85. https://doi.org/10.1016/j.gene.2019.01.048.

39. M. L. Ahui et al., "Ginger Prevents Th2-Mediated Immune Responses in a Mouse Model of Airway Inflammation," *International Immunopharmacology* 8, no. 12 (2008): 1626–32. https://doi.org/10.1016/j.intimp.2008.07.009.

40. R. Borenstein et al., "Ginkgolic Acid Inhibits Fusion of Enveloped Viruses," *Scientific Reports* 10, no. 1 (2020): 4746. https://doi.org/10.1038/s41598-020-61700-0.

41. H. Woelk et al., "Ginkgo Biloba Special Extract EGb 761® in Generalized Anxiety Disorder and Adjustment Disorder with Anxious Mood: A Randomized, Double-Blind, Placebo-Controlled Trial," *Journal of Psychiatric Research* 41, no. 6 (2007): 472–80. https://doi.org/10.1016/j.jpsychires.2006.05.004.

42. M. M. Villaseñor-García et al., "Effect of Ginkgo Biloba Extract EGb 761 on the Nonspecific and Humoral Immune Responses in a Hypothalamic-Pituitary-Adrenal Axis Activation Model," *International Immunopharmacology* 4, no. 9 (2004): 1217–22. https://doi.org/10.1016/j.intimp.2004.05.014.

43. K. I. Block and M. N. Mead, "Immune System Effects of Echinacea, Ginseng, and Astragalus: A Review,"

Integrative Cancer Therapies, September 2003: 247–67. https://doi.org/10.1177/1534735403256419.

44. Ibid.

45. G. Predy et al., "Efficacy of an Extract of North American Ginseng Containing Poly-Furanosyl-Pyranosyl-Saccharides for Preventing Upper Respiratory Tract Infections: A Randomized Controlled Trial," *CMAJ* 173, no. 9 (2005): 1043–48. https://doi.org/10.1503/cmaj.1041470.

46. C. A. Rowe et al., "Specific Formulation of *Camellia sinensis* Prevents Cold and Flu Symptoms and Enhances γδ T Cell Function: A Randomized, Double-Blind, Placebo-Controlled Study," *Journal of the American College of Nutrition* 26, no. 5 (2007): 445–52. https://doi.org/10.1080/07315724.2007.10719 634.

47. D. Furushima, K. Ide, and H. Yamada, "Effect of Tea Catechins on Influenza Infection and the Common Cold with a Focus on Epidemiological/Clinical Studies," *Molecules* 23, no.7 (2018): 1795. https://doi .org/10.3390/molecules23071795.

48. J. Xu, Z. Xu, and W. Zheng, "A Review of the Antiviral Role of Green Tea Catechins," *Molecules* 22, no. 8 (2017): 1337. https://doi.org/10.3390/molecules22081337.

49. M. T. Sultan et al., "Immunity: Plants as Effective Mediators," *Critical Reviews in Food Science and Nutrition* 54, no. 10 (2014): 1298–308. https://doi.org/10.1080/10408398.2011.633249.

50. T. Utsunomiya et al., "Glycyrrhizin, an Active Component of Licorice Roots, Reduces Morbidity and Mortality of Mice Infected with Lethal Doses of Influenza Virus," *Antimicrobial Agents and Chemotherapy* 41, no. 3 (1997): 551–56. https://doi.org/10.1128/AAC.41.3.551.

51. Y. Yang et al., "Traditional Chinese Medicine in the Treatment of Patients Infected with 2019-New Coronavirus (SARS-CoV-2): A Review and Perspective," *International Journal of Biological Sciences* 16, no. 10 (2020): 1708–17. https://doi.org:/10.7150/ijbs.45538.

52. J. Cinatl et al., "Glycyrrhizin, an Active Component of Liquorice Roots, and Replication of SARS-Associated Coronavirus," *Lancet* 361, no. 9374 (2003): 2045–46. https://doi.org/10.1016/s0140 -6736(03)13615-x.

53. G. Pastorino et al., "Liquorice (*Glycyrrhiza glabra*): A Phytochemical and Pharmacological Review," *Phytotherapy Research* 32, no. 12 (2018): 2323–39. https://doi.org/10.1002/ptr.6178.

54. V. Somerville, R. Moore, and A. Braakhuis, "The Effect of Olive Leaf Extract on Upper Respiratory Illness in High School Athletes: A Randomised Control Trial," *Nutrients* 11, no. 2 (2019): 358. https://doi .org/10.3390/nu11020358.

55. T. Magrone et al., "Olive Leaf Extracts Act as Modulators of the Human Immune Response," *Endocrine, Metabolic & Immune Disorders—Drug Targets* 18, no. 1 (2018): 85–93. https://doi.org/10.2174/1871530 317666171116110537.

56. American Chemical Society, "Researchers Call Herbs Rich Source of Healthy Antioxidants; Oregano Ranks Highest." *ScienceDaily*, January 8, 2002. www.sciencedaily.com/releases/2002/01/020108075158.htm.

57. E. P. Gutiérrez-Grijalva et al., "Flavonoids and Phenolic Acids from Oregano: Occurrence, Biological Activity and Health Benefits," *Plants* 7, no. 1 (2017): 2. https://doi.org/10.3390/plants7010002.

58. P. Kubatka et al., "Oregano Demonstrates Distinct Tumour-Suppressive Effects in the Breast Carcinoma Model," *European Journal of Nutrition* 56, no. 3 (2017): 1303–16. https://doi.org/10.1007/s00394-016 -1181-5.

59. Z. E. Suntres, J. Coccimiglio, and M. Alipour, "The Bioactivity and Toxicological Actions of Carvacrol," *Critical Reviews in Food Science and Nutrition* 55, no. 3 (2015): 304–18. https://doi.org/10.1080/104083 98.2011.653458.

60. N. Bhardwaj, P. Katyal, and A. K. Sharma, "Suppression of Inflammatory and Allergic Responses by Pharmacologically Potent Fungus Ganoderma lucidum," *Recent Patents on Inflammation & Allergy Drug Discovery* 8, no. 2 (2014): 104–17. https://doi.org/10.2174/1872213x08666140619110657.

61. W. Tang et al., "Ganoderic Acid T from *Ganoderma lucidum* Mycelia Induces Mitochondria Mediated Apoptosis in Lung Cancer Cells," *Life Sciences* 80, no. 3 (2006): 205–11. https://doi.org/10.1016/j.lfs.2006.09.001.

62. M. M. Martínez-Montemayor et al., "Ganoderma lucidum (Reishi) Inhibits Cancer Cell Growth and Expression of Key Molecules in Inflammatory Breast Cancer," *Nutrition and Cancer* 63, no. 7 (2011): 1085–94. https://doi.org/10.1080/01635581.2011.601845.

63. N. Bhardwaj, P. Katyal, and A. K. Sharma, "Suppression of Inflammatory and Allergic Responses by Pharmacologically Potent Fungus Ganoderma lucidum," *Recent Patents on Inflammation & Allergy Drug Discovery* 8, no. 2 (2014): 104–17. https://doi.org/10.2174/1872213x08666140619110657.

64. M. Ahmed et al., "*Rhodiola rosea* Exerts Antiviral Activity in Athletes Following a Competitive Marathon Race," *Frontiers in Nutrition* 2, no. 24 (2015). https://doi.org/10.3389/fnut.2015.00024.

65. Y. Li et al., "*Rhodiola rosea* L.: An Herb with Anti-Stress, Anti-Aging, and Immunostimulating Properties for Cancer Chemoprevention," *Current Pharmacology Reports* 3, no. 6 (2017): 384–95. https://doi.org/10.1007/s40495-017-0106-1.

66. K. F. Benson et al., "The Mycelium of the *Trametes versicolor* (Turkey Tail) Mushroom and Its Fermented Substrate Each Show Potent and Complementary Immune Activating Properties in Vitro," *BMC Complementary and Alternative Medicine* 19, no. 1 (2019): 342. https://doi.org/10.1186/s12906-019-2681-7.

67. C. J. Torkelson et al., "Phase 1 Clinical Trial of *Trametes versicolor* in Women with Breast Cancer," *ISRN Oncology*, 2012, article 251632. https://doi.org/10.5402/2012/251632.

68. P. M. Kidd, "The Use of Mushroom Glucans and Proteoglycans in Cancer Treatment," *Alternative Medicine Review: A Journal of Clinical Therapeutics* 5, no. 1 (2000): 4–27. https://pubmed.ncbi.nlm.nih.gov/10696116.

69. A. Noorafshan and S. Ashkani-Esfahani, "A Review of Therapeutic Effects of Curcumin," *Current Pharmaceutical Design* 19, no. 11 (2013): 2032–46.

70. Ibid.

71. Ibid.

72. R. E. Carroll et al., "Phase IIa Clinical Trial of Curcumin for the Prevention of Colorectal Neoplasia," *Cancer Prevention Research* 4, no. 3 (2011): 354–64. https://doi.org/10.1158/1940-6207.CAPR-10-0098.

The Importance of Vitamins

1. P. W. Tebbey and T. M. Buttke, "Molecular Basis for the Immunosuppressive Action of Stearic Acid on T Cells," *Immunology* 70, no. 3 (1990): 379–84.

2. Z. Huang et al., "Role of Vitamin A in the Immune System," *Journal of Clinical Medicine* 7, no. 9 (2018): 258. https://doi.org/10.3390/jcm7090258.

3. C. Aranow, "Vitamin D and the Immune System," *Journal of Investigative Medicine* 59, no. 6 (2011): 881–86. https://doi.org/10.2310/JIM.0b013e31821b8755.

4. A. C. Carr and S. Maggini, "Vitamin C and Immune Function," *Nutrients* 9, no. 11 (2017): 1211. https://doi.org/10.3390/nu9111211.

5. M. Pan et al., "Inhibition of TNF-α, IL-1α, and IL-1β by Pretreatment of Human Monocyte-Derived Macrophages with Menaquinone-7 and Cell Activation with TLR Agonists in Vitro," *Journal of Medicinal Food* 19, no. 7 (2016): 663–69.

6. C. Cheng, S. Chang, and B. Lee, "Vitamin B6 Supplementation Increases Immune Responses in Critically Ill Patients," *European Journal of Clinical Nutrition* 60 (2006): 1207–13. https://doi.org/10.1038/sj.ejcn.1602439.

Consume Antioxidant- and Mineral-Rich Foods

1. H. Hemilä, "Zinc Lozenges and the Common Cold: A Meta-Analysis Comparing Zinc Acetate and Zinc Gluconate, and the Role of Zinc Dosage," *JRSM Open* 8, no. 5 (2017). https://doi.org/10.1177/2054270417694291.

2. D. Hulisz, "Efficacy of Zinc Against Common Cold Viruses: An Overview," *Journal of the American Pharmacists Association* 44, no. 5 (2004): 594–603. https://pubmed.ncbi.nlm.nih.gov/15496046.

3. A. J. te Velthuis et al., "Zn(2+) Inhibits Coronavirus and Arterivirus RNA Polymerase Activity in Vitro and Zinc Ionophores Block the Replication of These Viruses in Cell Culture," *PLoS Pathogens* 6, no. 11 (2010): e1001176. https://doi.org/10.1371/journal.ppat.1001176.

4. P. R. Hoffmann and M. J. Berry, "The Influence of Selenium on Immune Responses," *Molecular Nutrition & Food Research* 52, no. 11 (2008): 1273–80. https://doi.org/10.1002/mnfr.200700330.

5. Ibid.

Optimize Gut Health

1. K. James et al., "Distinct Microbial and Immune Niches of the Human Colon," *Nature Immunology* 21 (2020): 343–53. https://doi.org/10.1038/s41590-020-0602-z.

2. D. Zheng, T. Liwinski, and E. Elinav, "Interaction between Microbiota and Immunity in Health and Disease," *Cell Research* 30 (2020): 492–506. https://doi.org/10.1038/s41422-020-0332-7.

3. C. Gao et al., "Gut Microbe–Mediated Suppression of Inflammation-Associated Colon Carcinogenesis by Luminal Histamine Production," *American Journal of Pathology* 187, no. 10 (2017): 2323–36. https://doi.org/10.1016/j.ajpath.2017.06.011.

Proper Hydration Tips

1. Y. David et al., "Water Intake and Cancer Prevention," *Journal of Clinical* Oncology 22, no. 2 (2004): 383–85. https://doi.org/10.1200/JCO.2004.99.245.

2. M. D. Allen et al., "Suboptimal Hydration Remodels Metabolism, Promotes Degenerative Diseases, and Shortens Life," *JCI Insight* 4, no. 17 (2019): e130949. https://doi.org/10.1172/jci.insight.130949.

3. A. Kamath et al., "Antigens in Tea-Beverage Prime Human Vγ2Vδ2 T Cells in Vitro and in Vivo for Memory and Nonmemory Antibacterial Cytokine Responses," *Proceedings of the National Academy of Sciences* 100, no. 10 (2003): 6009–14. https://doi.org/10.1073/pnas.1035603100.

4. T. Bahorun, A. Luximon-Ramma, V. S. Neergheen-Bhujun, T. K. Gunness, K. Googoolye, C. Auger, A. Crozier, O. Aruoma, "The Effect of Black Tea on Risk Factors of Cardiovascular Disease in a Normal Population," *Preventive Medicine.* 54, Suppl (2012): S98–102. https://doi.org/10.1016/j.ypmed.2011.12.009.

Sleep Strategies

1. S. Dimitrov et al., "Gα$_s$-Coupled Receptor Signaling and Sleep Regulate Integrin Activation of Human Antigen-Specific T Cells," *Journal of Experimental Medicine* 216, no. 3 (2019): 517–26. https://doi.org/10.1084/jem.20181169.

2. N. F. Watson et al., "Transcriptional Signatures of Sleep Duration Discordance in Monozygotic Twins," *Sleep* 40, no. 1 (2017): zsw019. https://doi.org/10.1093/sleep/zsw019.

3. A. A. Prather et al., "Behaviorally Assessed Sleep and Susceptibility to the Common Cold," *Sleep* 38, no. 9 (2015): 1353–59. https://doi.org/10.5665/sleep.4968.

4. S. Cohen et al., "Sleep Habits and Susceptibility to the Common Cold," *Archives of Internal Medicine* 169, no. 1 (2009): 62–67. https://doi.org/10.1001/archinternmed.2008.505.

Things to Avoid

1. L. A. Myles, "Fast Food Fever: Reviewing the Impacts of the Western Diet on Immunity," *Nutrition Journal* 13, article 61 (2014). https://doi.org/10.1186/1475-2891-13-61.

2. A. Christ et al., "Western Diet Triggers NLRP3-Dependent Innate Immune Reprogramming," *Cell* 172, no. 1-2 (2018): 162–75.e14. https://doi.org/10.1016/j.cell.2017.12.013.

3. D. Sarkar, M. K. Jung, and H. J. Wang, "Alcohol and the Immune System," *Alcohol Research: Current Review* 37, no. 2 (2015): 153–55. https://www.ncbi.nlm.nih.gov/pmc/articles/PMC4590612/; G. Szabo and B. Saha, "Alcohol's Effect on Host Defense," *Alcohol Research: Current Reviews* 37, no. 2 (2015): 159–70. https://www.ncbi.nlm.nih.gov/pmc/articles/PMC4590613/.

4. J. J. Milner and M. A. Beck, "The Impact of Obesity on the Immune Response to Infection," *Proceedings of the Nutrition Society* 71, no. 2 (2012): 298–306. https://doi.org/10.1017/S0029665112000158.

5. D. C. Nieman and L. M. Wentz, "The Compelling Link between Physical Activity and the Body's Defense System," *Journal of Sport and Health Science* 8, no. 3 (2019): 201–17. https://doi.org/10.1016/j.jshs.2018.09.009.

6. D. C. Nieman et al., "Upper Respiratory Tract Infection is Reduced in Physically Fit and Active Adults," *British Journal of Sports Medicine* 45, no. 12 (2011): 987–92. https://doi.org/10.1136/bjsm.2010.077875.

7. S. Cohen et al., "Chronic Stress, Glucocorticoid Receptor Resistance, Inflammation, and Disease Risk," *Proceedings of the National Academy of Sciences* 109, no. 16 (2012): 5995–99. https://doi.org/10.1073/pnas.1118355109.

Note: Page numbers in *italics* indicate recipes;
page numbers in **bold** indicate main listing and definition.
Page numbers in parentheses indicate intermittent references.

ABOUT THE AUTHOR

Dr. Joseph Mercola is a physician and *New York Times* best-selling author. He was voted the Ultimate Wellness Game Changer by *The Huffington Post* and has been featured in several national media outlets, including *Time* magazine, the *Los Angeles Times*, CNN, Fox News, ABC News, *TODAY*, and *The Dr. Oz Show*. He founded his website, mercola.com, in 1997 well before Google, Amazon, and Facebook, and it has been the most visited natural health site on the web for the last 15 years.

Website: Mercola.com

Hay House Titles of Related Interest

YOU CAN HEAL YOUR LIFE, the movie, starring Louise Hay & Friends
(available as a 1-DVD program, an expanded 2-DVD set, and an online streaming video)
Learn more at www.hayhouse.com/louise-movie

THE SHIFT, the movie,
starring Dr. Wayne W. Dyer
(available as a 1-DVD program, an expanded 2-DVD set, and an online streaming video)
Learn more at www.hayhouse.com/the-shift-movie

***

ALCHEMY OF HERBS, by Rosalee de la Forêt

CANCER-FREE WITH FOOD, by Liana Werner-Gray

FAT FOR FUEL KETOGENIC COOKBOOK, by Dr. Joseph Mercola and Pete Evans

KETOFAST COOKBOOK, by Dr. Joseph Mercola and Pete Evans

***

All of the above are available at your local bookstore,
or may be ordered by contacting Hay House (see next page).

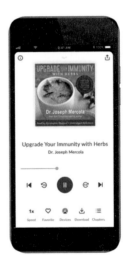

Free e-newsletters from Hay House, the Ultimate Resource for Inspiration

Be the first to know about Hay House's free downloads, special offers, giveaways, contests, and more!

 Get exclusive excerpts from our latest releases and videos from *Hay House Present Moments*.

 Our *Digital Products Newsletter* is the perfect way to stay up-to-date on our latest discounted eBooks, featured mobile apps, and Live Online and On Demand events.

 Learn with real benefits! *HayHouseU.com* is your source for the most innovative online courses from the world's leading personal growth experts. Be the first to know about new online courses and to receive exclusive discounts.

 Enjoy uplifting personal stories, how-to articles, and healing advice, along with videos and empowering quotes, within *Heal Your Life*.

Sign Up Now!

Get inspired, educate yourself, get a complimentary gift, and share the wisdom!

Visit www.hayhouse.com/newsletters to sign up today!

 HAY HOUSE

 HAY HOUSE online learning